Thanks for the Mammaries

A Breast Cancer Survivor's Story

Sarah Demmon

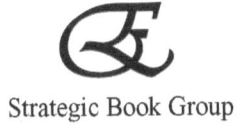

Strategic Book Group

Strategic Book Group
P.O. Box 333
Durham CT 06422
www.StrategicBookClub.com

ISBN: 978-1-60976-148-6

Printed in the United States of America

Book Design: Suzanne Kelly

Dedication

THIS BOOK IS DEDICATED to the millions of people diagnosed with breast cancer as they embark on the battle of their lives.

Acknowledgements

FIRST, I HAVE TO GIVE PROPS to Kristi who simply said, "You have to take these emails and make them into a book." I want to thank all the fabulous doctors and nurses in the Clarian Health system in Indianapolis. I want to especially thank Dr. Bryan Schneider, my oncologist, and his fabulous clinical nurse Danielle who both continue to put up with my non-compliant ass, incessant questions and surly attitude. Finally, I have to give a shout out to all my peeps for taking care of me and getting me through this little bump in the road.

Table of Contents

Introduction

'YOU HAVE BREAST CANCER.' These four words have been uttered to the famous, the rich, the poor and to me in August of 2007. This statement has the power to make a person experience fear, depression and anxiety all in one moment. You want to know why this is happening to you and what you have done so wrong in your life to deserve this diagnosis. The human brain is an amazing organ that is normally so useful, but in times like these, the brain can turn on you and bring about images of yourself as a cancer patient, bald and gaunt, lying in a pool of your own vomit with death surely to follow. If you are a fellow traveler on the breast cancer journey, then let me tell you that while that image of a cancer patient may have been true years ago, it is not necessarily true now—well except for the baldness. While no two stories are alike, maybe you will find within mine a small lesson that I learned that you will benefit from when faced with a similar situation and will know what to do through my guidance. When I was searching for facts to help prepare me for the experience I was about to embark on, all I could find was a lot of touchy, feely books and websites that were testimony to the emotion of the disease, but said little of the factual experience. I only wanted to know what to do first. I wanted a one-stop resource that had cold, hard facts. I would like to think that I am helping ease the start of someone else's journey.

Before you get into my story, I have to warn you that this narrative is brutally honest, and contains some foul language, much like watching an episode of Kathy Griffin, who, by the way, is a kick-ass comedian who offers comedic relief in any type of situation, as I hope this narrative will for those who are brave enough to continue. If you can get over my propensity to cuss like a sailor, then you will hopefully find something worthwhile in the contents of these pages. This book is really for those who do not deal with the curve balls that life throws at them in the overtly emotional manner. Hey, if that approach works for you, great. For me, I am a take charge, independent sort of gal whose motto is "there is no crying at work," so why should there be crying about a little tumor. Okay there was some crying, but mostly a lot of drinking and swearing. I want to provide some facts interspersed with comic relief for those of us who, when faced with similar obstacles, say 'Fuck it,' and tackle it with gusto. Frankly, I have yet to find a source that has provided such information.

Now let me, in a non-self serving way, try to explain a little about myself before the cancer. I grew up in a small Indiana town, in an area that is known as 'The Region,' located at northwest Indiana, close to Chicago. I graduated from Butler University with a degree in Chemistry, received a Master's degree in Biochemistry from Purdue, but I am a fan of Purdue's archrival, Indiana University. So there is a great deal of confusion in my life when the basketball season, a religious time in Indiana, comes. I love to do all sorts of sports and to be outside, in general. I am also a research scientist—with a fabulous pocket protector—and would like to think, without being arrogant, that I do my job well, largely due in part to my overwhelming talent—okay just kidding, I am a workaholic. I am the type of employee who comes in sick and contaminates others. This is mostly because I do not like to lie around and I find that daytime TV sucks. To date, I have not been married—this is beginning to sound like a personal ad . . . I also like puppies, pina coladas and getting caught in the rain—nor to date had kids, but I am an aunt or pseudo aunt to many. I am very driven in everything that I do. This can be good and bad, in that my competitiveness sometimes leads me to not let the seven-year-olds win at Candy Land. All of the above traits are necessary to know in order to understand my point of view with this story.

Another big impetus for documenting my cancer adventures was for me mostly attributed to the fact that around every corner there was an unexpected surprise, whether it was knowing what to do next, dealing with doctors, not realizing the cost of being sick or just if what I was feeling was okay. This was because nothing with this disease seemed to be straight forward. For a data driven girl like myself, it is the most disheartening, cruel part of the disease. If I can at least provide information to the average person going through this, then maybe I am doing my job. If not, at least I can provide some humor on a humorless situation. At the end of most days, laughter is what got me through it, or at least it took the edge off my frustrations.

Your Support System: A Couple of Jack Assess and No Whiners

EXCERPT FROM AN EMAIL, 8/28/2007:

"I would hope that you all would continue to harass me as you normally would. You all know my sense of humor and will act accordingly."

No matter how independent you think you are, you cannot go through this alone. Whether it is a spouse, significant other, or friend, you need someone to go through this with you. My single ass needed to either find a dude who dug bald chicks really quick, or rely on my family and friends. In my case, the majority of my care was administered by my best friend, due to the fact that she lives just the next street over.

Let me tell you about the kind of friends that you need: You need your true homies—the ones that will not give your pathetic ass any room to feel sorry for yourself, because you are going to go down that road many times. My best friend Lindsey is a jackass just like I am. I do say this proudly. How much of a jackass is she, you may ask? Let me give an example. Two months after my father died, a group of us decided to go to Oprah. One of our friends lived in Chicago at the time, so we were making a weekend of it. We were psyched because it takes forever to get Oprah tickets. We showed up hoping it was going to be one of the shows where you leave with a bunch of cool free shit. Well,

1

we sat down and the producer came out to announce the topic of the show.

"Ladies and Gentlemen, today's topic is a serious one. We will be discussing death and dying."

I turned to my friends with a look that said, "Oh shit, this is just great."

They proceeded with the show about these people who were dying and how they were preparing themselves and their families. About twenty minutes into the show, I was weeping uncontrollably. Instead of consoling me, Lindsey proceeded to yell at me for the way I was wiping my eyes. She said, "Demmon, what the hell are you doing? You are smearing your make up. You see, you must gently sweep upwards underneath the eyes so as not to mess up the makeup, don't you know?"

I could give countless other examples, but again, that may be another book.

Lindsey and I met in college as we both ran cross country for Butler University. She was studying to be a pharmacist and I was in the chemistry program. It was an auspicious beginning—starting with exercise and eventually morphing into partying. I ended up in the same sorority because of her recruitment. Later she told me, "Misery loves company." I wish I had known her game earlier. I have been friends with both her and her husband for over twenty years. We have been through her having kids, me losing my father and the general rigors of life. However, I cannot say that those experiences were what enabled me to get through this.

I also attribute my resolve to years and years of sports. Where else do you push yourself to such physical and mental limits on a regular basis and come back for more? My friends and I have had several discussions on our approach to life's issues, and sports seems to always come back as the answer for most of our resolve. Not that I am saying that sports has made me so self reliant that I thumb my nose at society and breezed through this all by myself. I will admit that it is through the grace of God, through Lindsey's support, and the support of others that I have maintained my sense of self throughout this ordeal. Lindsey's sense of reality and honesty provided the most comfort during this ordeal, not "Do you need a hug?" I know that works great for some, but like I mentioned earlier, I am not that kind of person. As one of my closest friends, she knew that was not what I needed as an initial approach. In fact it became a running joke that we would ask each other 'Do you need a hug?'

On the other hand, people were telling Lindsey that she could not take the pressure of having to support my ass and was going to break down. This would just piss her off further. The funny thing in all this is that not once did anyone say that to me. Hey, I was the one who was sick!

Another of my best friends, Cindy, with whom I happen to work with, is a firm believer in tough love as well. She often would yell at me for working when I should have been at home, yet she did not coddle me when I felt bad. The fact that I chose to surround myself with these personality types points to my own sadistic nature, but at least our conversations are never dull and we challenge each other daily. I am a huge believer that attitude is everything and I do not subscribe to reveling in the shittiness of a situation. Those closest to me know this and made sure that when I was down and hurting, they were consistent in their message—this is just a small moment to get to the end point. When I was negative, they were positive, no matter the subject: loss of boobs, feeling like ass, balding like Kojak, etc.

What you do not need is people who are negative or are wallowers. By wallowers I mean they want to revel in the glory of your grief and make it their own. They become consumed by your disease and the drama is more satisfying to them than the lifetime movie of the week. They will suck you down with them into a pit of despair that will involve hugging and crying every time they see you. They want to share their own personal stories of cancer that inevitably lead to the death or horrible suffering of the individual they speak about—always uplifting to you as you listen. And of course they give you the look. The look, which you get from complete strangers when you go out in public, involves a slight tilt to the head, a downward cast to the eyes and a gaze that condemns you to death. It is the look of pity and sorrow

3

that you do not feel until someone gives you the look. You are be-bopping around just fine, feeling pretty good about yourself, until you get 'the look.' I have been told I am not allowed to slap anyone that gives me the look, but it is very tempting. The irony of it all is that usually those giving you the look are fucked up themselves. I got the look from a chick at Blockbuster wearing fuzzy pink slippers. Who the fuck wears fuzzy pink slippers to rent a movie? Another violator was a chick who obviously had spent way too much time in the tanning bed. I felt like saying, "Yes, I have breast cancer, but you are well on your way to skin cancer which, by the way, you ignore that is the largest organ of your body—good luck with that!"

Sorry about my mini Dennis Miller rant, it just needed to be addressed.

Back to your support system. What you do not realize is that as much as you do not want to, whoever you choose to rely on, you are going to have to get over the guilt of stressing them out. It is not in my nature to cause others stress or grief. I would like to think of myself as someone who relieves stress—someone who others rely on. I can tell you that for me it is a strange place to become reliant on others. You must have someone that you absolutely trust with your life because there will be times when you will be in a place where you need someone to take over. You must trust in your relationship with your support personnel and that they can handle the stress of your disease on top of the normal stresses of daily life without resenting you. This truly got tested during my ordeal. I remember one of the first nights after getting diagnosed, I was sitting on my deck with Lindsey and I said to her, "You are going to have to let me know if this gets too much because I am going to have to rely on you to get me through this. You have three kids and a life to live as well. I don't want to cause a lot of extra stress to your already stressful life."

She accepted this challenge without a blink of an eye. I knew she would, but I felt like I had to verbalize the situation for myself, if nothing else, because I was in unfamiliar territory. My previous independence was going to be gone in an instance. To top all this off, soon after getting diagnosed, another close friend, Ginger, was diagnosed with myasthenia gravis, a disease that causes severe weakness of the muscles. Treatment for the disease could be anywhere from several months to years. Her ordeal could be a separate book. Lindsey was now faced with having two good, life-long friends facing life-altering diseases.

Lindsey joked, "Demmon, I think I have survivor's guilt."

In a way, Ginger's disease allowed me to fly under the radar as she also has three kids and needed more support than myself. I preferred to have the attention diverted away from my plight as I tend to suffer in silence. I am one of those people who when they are sick, just want to be left alone. That being said, they knew when not to leave me alone. It also was definitely the sick sense of humor that we all share that kept us with our heads above water. Regardless, every time I needed to ask for help, it was painful for me to do, but I realized that I was asking for help because I really needed it. At the start of all this, Lindsey and I were walking away from one of my first doctor's appointments and I turned to her and jokingly said, "I always thought that you would take care of my kids someday, as I have with yours, but never imagined in a million years that you would need to take care of me instead."

The Lump:
"Yo Doc, Somethin' Ain't Right"

PRIOR TO THIS ORDEAL I had never had a serious illness. I had never had surgery, never a major broken bone and never had stayed in the hospital overnight. I cannot tell you when the lump made its debut. I was not a regular self exam person, because I have very dense, fibrous breasts, which all but makes a self exam impossible. It is like feeling two sacks full of bb pellets—I will never be Danielle Steele, "as he ripped off her shirt and ran his hands over her voluptuous sacks of bb pellets . . . " Because of the lumps and bumps, I was not concerned about the lump at first. My mother also has fibrocystic breasts, further helping to rationalize in my brain the lumps in my breasts were nothing up until the day I was biopsied. Here is where the system begins to break down. I had been going yearly for a physical as my doctor requires them to remain as his patient. Let me interject here that I like this doctor very much. He always takes time at the beginning of every appointment to talk to me as a human being, discussing what has gone on over the past year and how I have felt. He has always been thorough in his exams in discussing blood work and lifestyle habits to remain healthy. I am still his patient to this day.

Part of that physical is his examination of the girls. He would always comment on the lumps and bumps, but never seemed concerned. The funny thing is that the doctor would always ask if I was concerned about the lumps and I would answer, "No," because he was not worried, so why should I be?

Looking back, I wonder why he would ask me this. I am a chemist, not a doctor—but I did stay in a Holiday Inn Express.... To his credit, the statistics were on his side. I had no family history of breast cancer; I was under thirty years old and was very healthy. At the age of thirty-five, the doctor ordered my baseline mammogram, which is typical. So off I went to one of the most pleasant experiences in a female's life: the squishing of the boobs. I am confident a man has to have invented the mammogram—squeezing the living shit out of your boobs. I am sorry, but they were never meant to be flattened in such a manner. The mammogram typically is performed at an imaging center, separate from the doctor's office. You do not see a doctor there, but instead a technician and possibly a radiologist to talk to you about your films. The procedure involves you standing shirtless in front of a machine. The technician will place your breast in the apparatus and slowly clamp down on it. My advice is to not look down.

The technician will then tell you, "Don't breathe."

I thought, "Don't worry; I can't because I think you put part of my lung in the machine."

After taking standard images, they may ask you to wait to take additional images if the radiologist is not happy with the first set of films.

Two days after my first mammogram, I got the phone call that I needed to come back for more images. I freaked out initially, but when I talked to my mom, I found out that this was a phone call she got all the time, so I felt a little better. When I returned to experience the mammogram again, they focused on the right side and indicated that I had calcium deposits they wanted to monitor. Looking back, if I knew then what I know now, I would have insisted on an ultrasound or magnetic resonance imaging (MRI.). What I found out during the course of all this is that if you have dense breasts, the only thing the mammogram is good for is seeing calcium deposits but is not so good for seeing tumors in dense breasts. Calcium deposits can be indicative of cancer. Calcium deposits can also surround fibroids, so for women like me with dense breasts, there is no absolute way to tell why you have them in your breast, other than going to other imaging techniques. The very important lesson learned is that if you have been told you have dense breasts; do not fuck around with mammograms. Get the MRI or ultrasound.

After that mammogram, I became conscious of the lump for the first time. I could feel it lurking under the skin. When I first felt it, the lump seemed to be about the size of an olive. The lump was visible through the skin and became something that would throb during premenstrual period. I did tell the doctor about this, but it was another sign that was missed. The majority of breast cancers that are diagnosed feed off of the estrogen in our body. The fact that it would flare up during peak estrogen times in my cycle was another small, yet significant sign that I should have pointed out to my doctor during routine exams. I found out later from the doctor that the lump could have been there for five to ten years. That little piece of trivia was sort of shocking to me, especially with all the imaging that I had performed before the diagnosis.

After my first set of mammograms at the age of thirty-five, I was told that they would monitor the calcium deposits with a follow up mammogram in six months. Nothing was said about the lump. I went about my business with no second thought. At each subsequent follow-up mammogram, I would let them know about my fibrous breasts and the lump, but no one seemed concerned. My regular doctor would ask me if I was concerned about the lump. Here is where, looking back, I feel that was a very unfair question to ask me. I am not the doctor, and frankly, if the doctor does not look or act concerned, then why should I be freaking out? I am not a hypochondriac. I do not go through life constantly thinking something is wrong with me. In fact, if you ask my friends, I hate going to the doctor. I was raised under the motto of 'suck it up.' Being the athlete that I am, I am frequently getting injured and probably should go to the doctor for the injuries, yet in most cases, I do not. At my physical I had right before being diagnosed, I was asked again if I was concerned about the lump.

I asked the doctor, "Are you concerned?"

He answered, "It is probably nothing, given your mom's history. I tell you what, why do we not schedule an appointment to see a breast surgeon, if nothing else for cosmetic reasons, since the lump is protruding."

Had the lump not been visible and had it not been so painful during the premenstrual period, I probably would have never vocalized any concern to my doctor.

Before the visit to the surgeon, I went off for my annual boob squishing. I was going every six months, but had graduated to a year. As I had every other time, I showed off my lump and submitted for my usual pleasantries. After completion of the mammogram imaging, the technician and the radiologist on-site that reads the images came into the room and said they were taking me to perform an ultrasound. This was new. She proceeded to drag me into another room and started scanning my breast. The radiologist started making comments about the lump and the tone of the conversation was not comforting.

I asked, "What is going on?"

Instead of explaining things to me as a human, the on-site doctor started bitching me out about the lump.

The technician asked, "How long have you had this?" Followed by, "Have you told anyone about this lump?"

I started to get a little pissed. When I am attacked, I tend to go on the offensive verbally, and so I was trying very hard not to start chewing these people a new asshole. I was there by myself and was made to feel like I had done something wrong. Well, I find this a common theme when I work with doctors and something does not go right.

I said, "Look, I have been telling this office about the lump ever since my first mammogram. Just tell me what I need to do to get this resolved."

They wanted me to get a biopsy right away. I was sent to a surgeon who is well known in the area. A friend had been treated by him and loved him. When I called for the appointment, I could not get in to see him, but was instead given one of his associates. I asked before going if I needed a driver and was told I did not. So I show up thinking that this was going to be something like getting blood drawn. I was *wrong*.

Not once was the procedure explained to me. I hopped on the table and the associate entered. He explained his near brush with chemistry as a career expecting me to be impressed. I feigned interest as I was thinking, "Gee, I hope you did all right in chemistry as it is a big part of your core courses."

He then explained they were going to numb the boob and stick a needle in and take a core sample of the lump.

Simple enough, right?

Wrong!

I reclined on my side in as casual a position as one can take with their boobs hanging out and wait for the numbing. It never came. All of a sudden there was a huge piercing pain in my chest as they began the procedure. At this point, I could not move for fear of causing more damage. All I could do was to lay there, with tears streaming down my face as for the next fifteen minutes my boob was painfully cored out. I was shaking so bad I thought that maybe I was having a seizure. They also declined to mention that they gave me a shot of adrenalin to minimize the bleeding.

The main doctor came in and asked, "Are you okay, honey?"

I was screaming in my mind, "No I am not fucking okay."

He then asked, "Do you want to take a break?"

Again, my mind was raging, "Why, yes I do. Let's go for a beer and talk about what is wrong in the world, starting with the huge ass needle sticking out of my breast and the pain that is as bad as when I tore my ankle in college running cross country, shall we?"

Instead I replied, "Just get it over with." Then, I said, "You did not prepare me for this at all."

This fact did not seem to affect them.

Let me pause here to explain what they really do. They take these huge needles with big ass holes in them, and using ultrasound to guide placement, they stick them directly into your breast trying to get into the center of the lump. Because they use ultrasound, it is not a quick in and out procedure. They move slowly in and make sure they are where they are supposed to be. They may also at that time deposit a marker to help identify the lump for future scans. Do not worry, as the marker is not large enough to set off metal detectors at the airport. I did ask! My lump happened to be near the top of my boob. I can only imagine the torture if the doctor would have to go into the center of the breast for a sample.

Needless to say, two big holes and a lot of bruising later, I was finished with my little torture session and told that they would call me in a couple of days to give me the results. Shit, I did not even get a sucker, a 'sorry,' 'hope you are okay,' 'do we need to call someone,' etc. So, my shaky, bleeding, in pain ass got in my car, turned it on, flipped to a violent song and started slamming the steering wheel while releasing a stream of obscenities to combat the adrenaline accumulated artificially and naturally in the doctor's office. If anyone had happened to pass by, they would have thought I escaped from the psychiatric ward and would have possibly looked for a straight jacket nearby. Needless to say, I was not happy.

Diagnosis: "I Have What?"

EMAIL EXCERPT, 8/28/2007:

"To recap, I was diagnosed with breast cancer 2 weeks ago. I have undergone a series of screens, through a couple of doctors and am ready to attack this thing."

August 14, 2007 is a day that will be etched in my brain forever. It was the afternoon and another exciting day at work of saving lives and making a difference when the phone rang. Caller identification indicated it was the hospital where I had the biopsy performed.

I picked up the phone with my usual cheery 'This is Sarah' which is code for 'What the fuck do you want?'

It was the junior doctor who started the conversation. He simply said, "We have the results from your biopsy and I am afraid that it appears to be breast cancer."

I replied, "Excuse me?"

There was dead silence on the phone, so I said, "Okay, do you know what kind?"

He indicated it was invasive ductile.

As my pulse began to reach light speed, I asked, "Umm can you tell me more?"

He replied, "Well, I would like you to come in and we can talk about it."

I jump on the offer with, "Do you have an appointment like now?"

"Well, I think I can fit you in tomorrow morning first thing," he said.

He then offered nothing else and just told me he would see me the following day. I can sum up how I was feeling in two words: HOLY SHIT. I immediately called Lindsey.

She and I do not typically talk to each other at work unless it is for a purpose, which is usually a request from her for me to pick up one of her kids. So she knew that I was not calling to idly chat about the day so far.

When she answered the phone, I started to really shake and I said "Hey Lindz, I just got a call from the doctor and he said I have breast cancer."

"What!?" she replied.

I repeated, "Yeah, he just called me and said I have invasive ductile cancer."

"Are you okay?" she asked.

"I don't know," I replied.

"I think you need to come home right now. Do you want me to come downtown and get you?"

"I will leave now, but I think I can drive myself home without killing anyone," I replied. I then called my boss, who was out of the office, and told her in one big sentence that I was just told I have breast cancer and I was going home. I think she was too stunned to ask questions and just said, "Okay."

I was barely holding it together at that point and very much wanted to vomit—which I subsequently did. I made it home without taking anyone out. I changed and went the next street over to Lindsey's house—we live half a mile away—and I remember walking in the door in a kind of numb haze. I cried some, but I could not really just let loose because I was just in a totally dazed state. I could tell that she was upset, which absolutely made me more upset because I knew that I caused it. I do not remember much from that evening as it was just kind of sitting around and letting it all sink in. There was no game plan at that point, other than Lindsey coming with me to the appointment. I called a couple other friends. Other than that, I did not talk to anyone. I could not physically do it. I can tell you this was night one of about seven in a row of multiple cocktails in the evening. You see my poison is Canadian Mist and Diet Sierra Mist. I funded both companies very well that week.

After the diagnosis, the first thing you want to do—which of course is the worst thing you can do—is hop your ass on the internet and figure out your condition. Within five minutes of surfing you will have convinced yourself that the tumor is in your brain and you are going to die in a week. I surfed for a whole ten minutes before I forcibly stopped myself, made a drink and went back to watching TiVo®. The internet, while being a great source of information for kids writing a report on Spain, has too much information and not enough cautions for the amateur physicians hopping on the electronic highway to self diagnosis. This is true of any medical mystery you are trying to solve for yourself, not just cancer. Hell, you could have a pain in your foot and by the end of a vigorous thirty minutes of surfing you will have convinced yourself that the pain is masking Lou Gehrig's disease and you better fill out the will.

Another fact I found after getting diagnosed with cancer was that everyone will tell you to go get Lance Armstrong's book. He is an athlete, I am an athlete—hey we have a lot in common, surely Lance will help me out. Hell to the no. Ninety percent of the book tells you how great Lance is and the other ten percent is about cancer, which is what you really want to know about, but not in enough detail to garner any worthwhile information. The first thing that Lance tells you is that he has the lung capacity of a mountain goat making him super human. Well that does not comfort the average individual who smoked in college. If it takes a world class athlete to beat cancer, then shit, I am screwed. I totally skipped the chapters about how great his wife was because if she was so great, then why was he screwing Sheryl Crow?

The information available for breast cancer takes on two types. The pure academic text books that contain loads of information but do not contain much insight, or the touchy, feely books that revel in the emotion of the disease, but contain no facts. The best way is to get a combination of books. I would like to say you have already made a great choice in selecting mine, but I would be remiss if I did not mention other references for situations that I cannot relate to like how to deal with your spouse, significant other or your children. One book that I really liked was "Be a Survivor" by Vladimir Lange. The book is short, not real in-depth, but contains nice synopses of various facts about the ordeal of breast cancer. What I found is that no source is one-stop shopping. The problem is that when you are diagnosed, the world becomes a whirlwind and you do not have the time to thoroughly research your situation. You want to stop the bus for a minute to gather your wits, but the driver ignores your pleas to pull over. In the end, I read very little and looked up things as I needed information. I would have loved to have had some insight that had real-life examples of what someone did in a particular situation. I guess in a society of lawsuits because you are not smart enough to drive without holding the hot coffee in your crotch, no source wants to give you a how-to approach. At the very least, I wanted a how-I-did-it approach, which is where Lance let me down. I do not mean to be so hard on Lance. It is just that my life could never compare to his, both physically and with respect to the resources at my disposal. At the end of this book, I have included a glossary of basic terms that you may hear and a list of questions that you may want to ask at various stages of your multiple visits to the doctor. Unlike a mullet, this book is a party in the front and business in the back.

The next morning, after the diagnosis, Lindsey and I showed up at the doctor's office. We were immediately escorted into a conference room. Unfortunately the path to the conference room involved walking past the staff who were all looking at us like they knew a train wreck was about to happen and they could not help but watch. As I think about it, it was the first time that people looked at me in a way that I was unaccustomed to: with pity. As we entered, there was a lone box of Kleenex sitting in the middle of the table.

Lindsey and I looked at each other, started laughing and said, "Well, I guess we aren't getting good news today."

Doctors pay attention and have a little tact. Subtly place the box of Kleenex in a place where you can pull it out if needed. As

I approached the conference table, I swept the box aside because I was there to get a game plan not fall apart.

The doctor starts in, "Sarah, you have invasive ductile cancer."

The word invasive strikes fear in anyone's heart. Let me be the first to tell you that all cancer is invasive. What matters is to what degree it has invaded. What the diagnosis meant in my case is that the cancer has spread to outside the duct. I explain this to the reader, because Shit Head did not explain this to me.

He then said, "There are several standard options for treatment. Given your age and state of health, I would say that you are probably going to have chemotherapy first, then surgery." He then began to explain about lumpectomies and mastectomies. I was still trying to process chemotherapy and he was going on about cutting things off. He topped this off with an explanation of the chances of recurrence based on the type of surgery you have. I was thinking, "I have not even dealt with what I have, let alone what could come back."

All the information that he had was based on reading a pathology slide. There will be no marker information as of yet. I will explain markers in a little bit. Remember this as you enter the office, that the doctor can only give you an overview at this point and will have very little specific information which is a big source of frustration for the patient as everything is moving at light speed.

Lindsey and I began to pepper the dude with questions. Junior had no idea what was about to come as the pharmacist and the chemist went to work on him.

"Let's back up a minute," I said. "Can we talk about the tumor? Do you know if it has spread anywhere?"

"No," he answered.

"You mentioned chemotherapy. Why would I do that first and not have the lump taken out right away?" I asked.

"Well, in my training…"

I immediately start screaming in my mind, "What?" In an effort to understand how this could have happened to me, I asked, "Do you know of a situation where a fibroid became cancerous?"

He replied, "Well anything is possible."

Lindsey replied, "That is not what she is asking. She is asking do you know of a situation where this has occurred?"

He insinuated that he had not heard of this happening. Lindsey then went on to ask how confident he was in the pathology findings and where he sent the slides. She knew of a previous situation at another hospital in Indianapolis where a patient was diagnosed with breast cancer and it turned out that the reading was false. The doctor began to take offense to our line of questioning. I could tell in his body language and his tone that he was no longer engaged.

I tuned him out after that. Lindsey was pelting him with questions, but I was shutting down. This guy was just spewing random facts and getting more and more defensive as we asked questions. He was not encouraging.

He never said, "This is how we are going to attack or fight." At this point, Lindsey picked up her purse off the floor. He realized then that we were over him.

He then said, "You are more than welcome to take this information for a second opinion."

Lindsey replied, "Yes we realize that. Thank you."

With that, we left his office.

What I realized later is that at that stage doctors are not able to tell you what you want to know because they do not know. What you want to know is: What kind?; Has it spread?; Is it slow or fast growing?; What's my prognosis?; How do I get rid of this?; etc. The only questions they can answer are the type and treatment.

All he had to say was, "I don't know, but we will find out this way."

I really don't think he expected the way we dealt with him. Instead of just sitting there and weeping, we challenged him to answer questions. Let me give you, doctors, another clue. If you do not know the answer to a patient's question, be honest. Do not speculate, do not make something up and most of all, do not turn it around to make the patient feel like they are incredibly stupid for asking the question or like they have done something wrong. We already feel like shit—no need to help out further. Besides, if patients are realistic, they will realize that you do not have all the answers. What the patient wants is a game plan to find out how to get those answers.

I left the office totally dejected. I walked out into the parking lot and tossed the keys to Lindsey. I had an overwhelming wave of depression come over me. I finally had my break down because my need to have data and a game plan was totally thwarted by the doctor's lack of energy towards my situation. Fortunately, having a friend who can take charge allowed me to not have to deal at that moment. When we got back to my house, Lindsey began calling her hospital connections, as she terms, her 'peeps.' I realize that not everyone will have the luxury of having these connections. If you do not, talk to people because what I found out is that most everyone has been touched either directly or indirectly by cancer. You can get a few names and hear about their experiences to evaluate who you should choose as your doctor. If you visit one of these doctors and you are not comfortable with them, keep looking. You are entitled to a second opinion. In fact, I encourage getting a second opinion. You will be spending a lot of time with this person, so you had better feel like you are in the best hands possible.

Here is the next lesson that I learned: Treating cancer involves a concert of doctors working together. There is no one-stop shopping with respect to doctors. You will need to find an oncologist, general surgeon and plastic surgeon. If you can, get doctors that are familiar with each other, because that is an even better situation. The oncologist manages your cancer treatment, while the surgeon manages your overall plan.

Lindsey called a surgeon that she knew was excellent. Unfortunately, I could not get into his office for three weeks. I could not wait that long. Being the control freak that I am, the thought of not having a game plan and not knowing if the cancer was localized or had spread throughout my body was killing me. Another surgeon with seventeen years of experience was recommended by a friend who is an anesthesiologist. She could get me in within the week, which was what my sanity needed. The surgeon is the first person you visit to get a game plan for your screening. By screening, I mean that you will go through a series of tests to determine the nature of your cancer.

That week of waiting I can honestly say was the longest week in my life and the most taxing one on my emotions. Every ache or pain immediately was translated to, "Oh, shit, that must be cancer too."

In the period of waiting I highly recommend finding someone to talk to that will give it to you straight. It will help your sanity while waiting for the results.

I called our friend Ann, who had breast cancer and a mastectomy a couple of years back. So, on a balmy late summer evening, I went over to her house with Lindsey. We sat in the back yard at their fabulous tiki hut, had a few beers and I bombarded her with questions. I chose to talk to Ann because I knew she would give me a straight story with no sugar coating. Talking to her helped validate the feelings I was having. By giving me a preview of what was to come, I was better prepared to deal with what might lie ahead. She was also a great example for me that I could come out on the other side of this okay. Anyone coming up to Ann off of the street could not tell that she was a cancer survivor. It gave me hope.

If you choose to go to another doctor than the one that originally diagnosed you, you will need to obtain your pathology slides before going, so that the second doctor can confirm the diagnosis. My first visit to the general surgeon confirmed that I had made the right choice in switching doctors. Unlike the Shit Head in diapers that spent twenty minutes with me,—I know, I am still a little angry. I guess I expected more—she spent over two hours with me to explain what she knew. She was honest when she did not know something, and laid out a game plan that was aggressive, fitting my state of mind. The plan was to start chemo first, followed by surgery entailing Sentinel Node Biopsy (SNB,) lumpectomy or possibly mastectomy, then radiation and finally, long-term therapy, depending on the outcome of marker testing. Markers tell you what type of tumor you have and are important in telling you what type of chemotherapy and long-term treatment you will receive.

Another thing you will need to know is that on top of all the shit you have to mentally process, if you are thinking about having kids, you may want to freeze some eggs away. I will dive into this a little more later, but when you come out of the other side of this, you may be menopausal, chemo may have damaged your eggs, or your treatment length may be such that when your body is ready again to have kids, you may decide it is not worth the risk because of age or your thoughts about what treatment might have done to your eggs. Just a little aside to add upon all the other glorious decisions you are about to embark upon.

The surgeon set up over the next week a game plan for getting information on the tumor. This would involve a breast MRI and a chest X-ray. I was also scheduled for a pelvic ultrasound as I had very heavy periods with occasional mid-cycle bleeding and a family history of ovarian cancer with my Grandmother on my Dad's side. This was the first time that I was told that a history of ovarian cancer also increases your risk for breast cancer. As I left the doctor's office, I could feel myself change modes. I went from a helpless person in the dark to someone with a plan to fight.

My first scheduled violation, I mean test, was the pelvic ultrasound. I had no idea what this entailed, but I assumed it would be similar to a normal ultrasound that you see people get all the time with the cold jelly on the belly. The first rain on that parade was when I was told I had to down 40 oz. of water two hours prior and could not pee. Apparently the bladder needs to be full for this test in order to image the organs better. I do not know how I made it to the exam without pissing my pants. My bladder was so painfully full I could have cried. When I stepped into the room there was the technician and a trainee. I was asked if I was okay with the trainee and I said I did not mind. I was then told to drop my pants to my knees and hop up on the table. And when I say pants, I mean both regular and underwear. I was not given a gown or anything. So I climbed up on the table with all my nether regions exposed for all to see. After a couple of minutes, the technician threw a towel over my nether regions and began the ultrasound. I felt like telling her not to bother. It was not like the free show had not already happened. The ultrasound took forever as the probe was pressed on my painfully full bladder. There was a lot of clicking on the image going on. I knew enough, having done microscopy at work, that she was measuring something. This started a panic that welled up in my chest. Holy shit, are those all tumors? To make matters worse, she declined to tell me what she was measuring. She was not allowed to tell me.

"Great. Where is my bottle of Xanax?"

Here is another learning point: When a pelvic ultrasound is performed, the technician takes many measurements of your internal organs for reference. That is what I was hearing the technician measure, not an army of tumors as my brain was imagining. It would have been nice for them to explain this to me but, as usual, I was left in the dark.

After completion of the pelvic ultrasound, I was given another treat I was not expecting: a vaginal ultrasound. I was asked to finally pee—more like I begged—and was then asked to gown up in a private room. Why in the hell did I not get to do that in the first place? Let me tell you that the vaginal ultrasound is a real great time. They roll a condom on the end of a big probe and violate you without dinner or a movie. Since the trainee was in the room, the technician would move the probe at odd angles and comment "see that?"

Again I was offered no explanation as to what they were talking about. Through all the initial tests, the best advice I can give is to wait to get your results from your doctor. Do not spend the entire time trying to read the technician's face for a sign of the test result. It will only serve to send you over the edge of the cliff you are so tenuously hanging on, then you will be driven to drink even more.

Following the pelvic ultrasound was the breast MRI. This involved lying on your stomach for thirty minutes with your hooters hanging below you. I did not mind it and fell asleep during the procedure. For the claustrophobic, however, lying in a tube where your arms are pinned to your sides because it is such a tight fit may bother you. The final coup de grace was the chest X-ray. This took all of two minutes. I can honestly say that any modesty I had was gone by the end of that week. I subsequently had no problem whipping any body part out to anyone that wanted a look or feel. In fact, I started contemplating charging ten dollars to feel the tumor to strangers on the street. I figured that was cheaper than what the prostitutes were offering on the East side of Indianapolis.

My next stop in the whirlwind tour of the medical community was to the oncologist. I had chosen to go to Indiana University Medical Center—the one thing I did get from Lance. The research hospital is top notch when it comes to treating cancer. I took my posse, Lindsey and Cindy, with me as I knew that I would be getting some results of my tests and to make sure that all the information that was presented was absorbed. Do not go to any doctor's appointments where information will be provided alone, especially in the early stages of your adventure. Unless you are a machine, you will never get all the information and you will walk out of the office forgetting to ask a question. There is power in numbers. To get into my oncologist was a two-hour wait, but well worth the time. The oncologist asked what I did for a living. I indicated that I was a research scientist. He then proceeded to tailor the conversation to my level of understanding. He first went through the diagnosis. I had a large tumor—5.5 cm measurement by hand—that appeared to be localized. There was no involvement in the other breast and the cancer did not appear to have spread to the lymph nodes as documented by MRI and physical exam. He then went on to explain the marker results. Tumors have markers that tell you information about their nature and give the doctor information for a course of treatment. The majority of breast cancers are estrogen receptor positive. This means that the tumor feeds off of the estrogen in your body. This explained the pain I had during peak times in my cycle—I always wanted the world to know about my cycle…. Another gene that is tested for is HER2. This is a normal receptor on the surface of the cell that is involved in cellular growth signaling pathways. In HER2 cancers, it is over expressed, meaning that the receptor is going wild, throwing a party and telling cells to grow inappropriately. While in the past, a HER2 positive diagnosis was not good, there have been recent advances in therapies that can target HER2 positive tumors. I was diagnosed with the common garden variety—estrogen receptor positive, HER2 negative. My hormones were having a kegger without my knowledge.

The rest of the news was a sigh of relief. My chest X-ray was negative as well as my pelvic ultrasound. This news coupled with the apparent lack of lymph node involvement meant that the party appeared to be contained. It is worth understanding that lymph node involvement cannot be absolutely determined until the time of surgery, and is called a sentinel node biopsy or SNB. Visually, my prognosis was as good as it could get. I felt immensely relieved. I then knew the enemy and it was not as daunting as it was in my worst imagination. Getting rid of it was going to try my resolve and kick my ass physically and mentally, but there was no reason why I could not get rid of it, which is what I was waiting to hear. The final piece to the oncologist's visit was to meet with my clinical nurse. My nurse, Danielle, was as cheeky as I was, so I knew that we would get along. She explained her role in my care. Any ache I had, any nausea, any sickness, any gut rot, etc. I was supposed to report to her imme-diately. She was to be my liaison to the oncologist. She sat down and gave me a whole wad of pamphlets ranging on a whole variety of subjects. There were the chemo pamphlets, which described the medicine and the side effects. There were also pamphlets for counseling. There was a leaflet describing local wig shops, and a prescription to go with it, that tailor to cancer survivors. Finally, there was a book and the best part of all, the free shit. Oh yes, there are perks to breast cancer. Those perks come in the form of free purses. Over the course of every doctor appointment, I would leave with something that was donated or another free purse. It was better than Oprah's free give-aways!

There are several courses of action which you will work out with your oncologist. Mine was chemo first, surgery later, then

23

radiation. The reason to do chemo first is to be able to see if your tumor will react to the course of treatment that is decided. If you start chemo and your tumor does not react, then the doctors can choose a different treatment regimen. If you take the lump out first, then you will have no idea if the treatment is actually working for your type of cancer. I was going to be put on a "dose-dense regimen," which means chemo every other week. Normally, chemo is every 3 weeks to give your body a little more time to recover in-between getting nuked. The dose-dense therapy is relatively new, but some studies have suggested that if the patient can tolerate the treatment, the long term prognosis was better than those on the conventional schedule.

Because of my young age and relative good health—except for a little cancer, I was healthy as a horse,—the more aggressive option was chosen. The standard treatment for estrogen receptor positive, HER2 negative cancer is ACT. Adriamycin/Cytoxan for four rounds, then four rounds of Taxol. What I did not realize about chemo is that for normal therapy, you are looking at five or six months. I guess I always thought it was a few doses and you were on your way. My timeline would be sixteen weeks of poisoning.

Too Much Information

EXCERPT FROM AN EMAIL, 10/4/2007:

"I am, by the way, charging $10 for anyone that wants to touch the tumor."

How much you choose to share with others is your choice. I chose to tell a few friends and to tell my work immediately after being diagnosed. Although I was sick and wrong, by that I mean, I made it very clear to my employers that I wanted to work throughout the process. I know some breast cancer survivors that had children took a whole year off, but for me, work provided a diversion from thinking about the disease. My job is such that I could work from home if needed. I am very lucky in that my place of work has been hugely supportive throughout the whole process. I continue to be overwhelmed to this day by the individuals who I have only briefly worked with that have reached out to offer support and genuinely mean it—Okay, so I have a little café mocha moment every now and then. I chose not to tell my family immediately, because there is a big difference in the following two phrases:

"Mom, I have cancer, but I don't know jack shit yet."

"Mom, I have cancer, but it is localized and treatable."

I just couldn't bear putting my mom through the wringer after all she had been through. My father passed away at the age of forty-eight from diabetes. My mom had to take care of him for the last four years of his life as he was incapacitated. He was already blind from the disease, making it that much harder. I knew that I was about to devastate her emotionally, and I just could not do it without being in a place where I knew what was going on. She was upset and disappointed that I did not come to her right away, but she seemed to get over it and saw my point. I chose to tell people in stages.

At work, I knew the rumor mill would start soon after I told a few individuals, so I then started what I called the 'cancer world tour.' There were certain people I wanted them to hear about it from my mouth instead of second hand. Again, a testament to my personality in that I was concerned about others' feelings over mine. Each day I would pick a few people, take them into a room and tell them the deal. I became very adept at delivering the news. My routine was pretty much like this:

"Hey, (insert informee's name here,) I just wanted you to hear this from me personally before you hear it from someone else. I was just diagnosed with breast cancer. I am doing okay, and you know I am too surly to let this bring me down." I would then start to joke to divert the heavy feeling in the room. The downside of delivering the same message over and over again is that I became calloused to the information and would forget that the person sitting across from me was hearing it for the first time. I would become momentarily confused as to why they were getting upset until I reminded myself that this was fresh to them. I can say that it was really the first time that I really realized the impact that I had on others and that they cared. I guess I do not really think about the amount of friends that I am truly blessed with. A problem of telling a large group of people that do care about your plight is then keeping them updated on every detail. I was not getting any work done because there were constantly people in my cubicle. It was then I made the decision to send email updates on a regular basis. Not quite a blog, but close. If anything, it was a good way to send the same piece of information to many. Since I was sending the information to people at work, I had to be careful with my wording. I never thought that my boobs would be a topic of work discussion, but at least I tried to make it tasteful. I was constantly thanked for being open and sharing with others. My readers clamored for more of my quick wit and open honesty.

You may not choose to be as open as I was and that is fine. You choose what you think others ought to know. In sending those emails, it was a way for me to let others know as well that I had not lost my sense of self. I infused in those emails the same sarcasm and attitude that I normally would impart in a conversation. In other words, the reader knew that I was okay. I have placed some of these emails throughout the book to give you a feel of the real time updates.

Chemo is Easy—It is Getting it in What is Hard

EMAIL EXCERPT FROM 10/4/2007:

"I apparently excel at everything, including clotting."

When you embark on the chemo journey, the first thing to tell yourself is that the experience is your own. It is good to ask around, but remember that how others tolerate the treatment will not be how you do. People, being the helpful souls that they are, will try to tell you that your experience will be horrible. They will tell some horror story of a friend of a friend who was miserable for the entire time. Do not listen to those stories. Again, let me interject that your mental state entering into chemo will help dictate how the course of your treatment runs. Make up your mind that you are entering into battle. I imagined that as the medicine entered my veins that it was ammunition flowing directly to the tumor. I truly believe that without buy in from the mind, the body will not be one hundred percent into the battle. Every time I went to treatment, I went with a positive attitude. I tried to do things afterwards like walking in the evening to make myself feel strong. Do everything you can to set yourself up for success. Also prepare yourself for the reality of feeling bad once in a while too. In other words, a tough mental attitude sprinkled with a dash of reality is the perfect formula for entering into chemo.

I began to hear about the side effects of chemo, besides losing your hair. There is a scary phrase called 'chemo brain.'

In a surprisingly large percentage of women, it was found that chemo makes them very scattered brained. The effect can be permanent or just last a few months, depending on the individual. This frightened the shit out of me considering how much I rely on memory and brain function to perform my job. I joked with Lindsey that my brains were my superpowers and I could not have them messed with. Fortunately, I experienced none of it—at least in my opinion, others may disagree—which I really attribute to the fact that outside of my normal work, I am constantly either working some sort of puzzle or reading. Much like physical exercise helps with the chemo, I am truly convinced that you need to do the mental exercising as well—I believe this to be true whether you are getting chemo or not: use it or lose it. If anything, exercising your mind by doing different tasks leads to more productivity other than pondering your disease state.

The one thing that makes chemo work is the exact thing that makes it tricky. It is nasty stuff and is designed to kill your cells. The medicine will trash your veins and thus it is recommended to have what is called a port which is surgically placed in a vein under your skin that allows for easy access for intravenous and blood draws. The port is basically a long catheter with an access site done surgically under MAC-sedation, which is a nice gentle anesthetic ride without being put completely under with a tube in your throat. The port can be placed in either your chest or under your arm along your side. This is usually determined by the doctor's preference in placement. The catheter is run through one of your major veins. Mine was put into my chest on the opposite side of the tumor. Some ports interfere with imaging, such as a MRI scan, so often they are put away from the cancer.

Five days before my first chemo appointment, I went in to surgery to have the port placed. Since you are receiving anesthetic, you cannot eat or drink at least twelve hours before the procedure. My surgery was scheduled for 2pm. Anyone that knows me is aware of two important facts. One, I drink a lot during the day, mostly some diet caffeinated beverage. Second, I can go without eating, but become even meaner than usual when my blood sugar dips. My tongue was stuck to the roof of my mouth by the afternoon, and any spit I could muster up was cherished as hydration by my body. I went to the hospital where Lindsey worked to have my port inserted. I was dropped off with the idea that she could then take me home when she got off of work. I lay in the pre-surgery room, patiently waiting for the time to go. This was my first ever surgery, so I was nervous. As 2pm approached, the nurse came in the room and indicated that my surgeon was tied up in another surgery, and was going to be late. The time kept creeping later and later. Finally at 5pm, the surgeon arrived. At this point, I was so miserable I could have cried. Lindsey along with the anesthesiologist wanted to reschedule. I was so pissed that I had to go through the day like this that I did not want to reschedule, because I felt like I had tortured myself all day for nothing. So they decided to go ahead. As they wheeled me down the hall, I passed Lindsey's pharmacy and raised my hands in the air with rock and roll fingers. She stepped out in her scrubs and started walking with the gurney.

"Where do you think you are going?" I asked.

"Demmon, I am going in," she replied.

"Great," I said. "Don't fuck anything up."

As we approached the operating room door, the nurse asked me if I wanted to walk into the room. I said, "Sure."

Then I heard Lindsey say, "Make sure you don't show them your junk."

I added another 'Fuck off' for good measure.

Lindsey ended up making an intravenous drip for me. I figured she would not let the help croak. I awoke in a pleasant, fuzzy haze. My evening was spent delightfully stoned from the after effects of the anesthetic. I was set to get my first infusion of poison.

Chemo day had arrived. Lindsey was my chemo buddy for the day. We went out for breakfast and then headed for the doctor's office. The routine for chemo is that you visit the oncologist first. My oncologist is very popular, so it was not uncommon to wait for up to two hours to see him. I learned after the first visit to schedule my appointment first thing in the morning before he got way behind. When the doctor finally does see you, he comes in, examines you and has blood drawn. This is your opportunity to speak with him on how you feel. It is very important to be honest. If you feel like shit, you should let the doctor know. The purpose of the blood draw is to make sure that your platelet level is high enough to withstand the assault on your body.

Once you are done with the oncologist, you are sent to the chemo lounge. You then have to sit and wait for a chair to open up, which could be another hour or so of waiting. The chemo lounge I visited consisted of two rooms with a bunch of recliners next to intravenous poles. The first visit is a shock. You can tell the newbies because they all have their hair. The lounge can be depressing if you allow it to be because there are some truly sick looking people in there. Always go with someone. The lounge has all types of people in there, not just breast cancer patients. There were men there as well, but most were well beyond my dating age range. Oh yes, I am shameless. A single girl is always looking for a date!

Technically I could have driven myself to chemo, but the experience is much more tolerable if you have someone to commiserate with. I made sure to spread the wealth so that one person was not burdened with taking me all the time. The other realization about chemo is that between the doctor visit and chemo, you are there all freaking day. Take a cooler of drinks at a minimum and maybe some snacks. I say maybe because the chemo lounge at the cancer center had a fabulous concept called the snack cart. There was always food available. At one chemo visit, I had to cut my friend Cindy off from the snack cart as she kept selecting various items at each pass. Of course none of it was for me, for fitness reasons.

The other issue to take in consideration regarding chemo is how you want to spend the day in treatment. I chose to take my iPOD® and laptop to do work. Others chose to nap. If you do not plan entertainment, then you are subjected to the random entertainment that can occur. The first time I showed up, the entertainment was the harp. No that is not a typo, there was a harp player. Now God bless the volunteers that come in and try to provide comfort, but here is how I see it from the patient's perspective: A harp reminds me of the music at a wake or a funeral. When I walked in with Danielle, my clinical nurse, I told her that she better put me in a different part of the lounge or at least get a shirtless Matthew McConaughey in to play the harp, otherwise, it sounded like a fucking funeral home and I wanted no part of it. You would think they would play more uplifting music, like "I Will Survive" or "Beat It." How about a stand-up comic to make people laugh? "A tumor walks into a bar..." Again, maybe I am not looking at things the right way. I have never claimed to be normal.

For the first four rounds, I was receiving two chemo drugs—Adriamycin and Cytoxan. What I describe next is the chemo regimen for my course of treatment. Other treatments will vary depending on the drugs that you are receiving. Before the chemo, you will receive an intravenous full of anti-nausea drugs that takes about fifteen minutes. Then, the Adriamycin is hooked up. The drug is red and you will consequently piss red for the next several hours. You will not want to have anything red to drink for a long, long time. This infusion also lasts about fifteen minutes. Now, there is a controversial issue about chewing ice or something cold during the infusion of Adriamycin. Apparently chewing ice during the infusion might reduce the incidence of mouth sores. My experience was that during the first infusion, I was too busy typing on my laptop to chew on it constantly and I had some pretty annoying sores on my tongue. For the remaining infusions, I was more diligent and began chewing ice. The amount of sores that I had was significantly less than before. So my vote is ice, ice baby. If you get the sores, there is an elixir called 'Mary's magic elixir' that can be prescribed to swish around in your mouth, that helps. It tastes really nasty, but does help. I found that Kanka, a brush with lidocaine, helped to numb the sore. It is available over the counter, and helped more than anything else.

During the same infusion time, following Adriamycin, they switch you to Cytoxan which can take anywhere from thirty minutes to an hour, based on your reaction to the drug. The Cytoxan can cause a runny, stuffy nose, so if you exhibit those symptoms, they will slow down the drip. My state of post nasal drip earned myself a forty-five minute infusion time. During my first chemo, I learned to drive. That is, after all those fluids being infused, I learned to move around the room to the bathroom while hooked up to an intravenous pole. I did run into a couple of people, but reassured them that I was a first time driver. I do not think they found this amusing, but my jack ass friend Lindsey was laughing hysterically from across the room. People were looking at us strangely. I could see what they were thinking.

"Who are these two idiots laughing while getting chemo? Can't they see this is a somber place? There's no laughing at chemo."

The misconception about chemo is that you are puking all the time and cannot eat. I found this to be quite the contrary for the chemo regimen required for breast cancer. They pump you so full of steroids—which also helps reduce the nausea—before and after, as well as other anti-nausea drugs, that you get so freaking hungry. The anti-nausea regimen that is available now is such that throwing up is rare. I did have bouts of nausea, but was able to manage it with medication. I was determined throughout the process not to gain weight. You see, the average person gains fifteen to twenty pounds on chemo. Hard to believe, but when you think about it, you are not nauseous so you continue to eat and you are tired so you lie about and do not work out. I gained about seven pounds.

After the first round of chemo I felt quite good, it only made me tired, mainly. When I got home, I had a headache and some dizziness. I would sleep a little, then get up and eat. Lindsey and I would try to walk as much as possible. A day after chemo, I had to do this shot of Neulasta that would allow my body to regenerate white blood cells quickly and pump up my immune system. When the shot kicks in,—about twenty-four hours after the shot—you are wiped out. It felt like every lymph node in my body was swollen. My skin was sore to the touch. All I could do was sleep to ride out the effects. You can imagine the delight at knowing what is about to transpire as you force yourself to give the shot. The importance of keeping my immune system up outweighed the day of misery that ensued after the shot. Another important thing to note is to keep away from sick people during chemo. You will be more susceptible than normal to getting a cold or the flu. You do not want to miss a treatment because some dumbass sneezed in your general direction.

My working out was cut short by all of my port fiascos. The story of port begins as follows. After my second round of chemo, I decided that I felt good enough to plant a tree. Lindsey came over as she decided, rightfully so, that I needed supervision for such a project. As I started digging, I came across a mean root system left from where I had pulled up a tree a couple of years ago. As thrilling as this narrative is, the stump plays a critical role in this story. I began to chop at the stump with a hatchet when I looked down at my left arm and realized that it had swelled up and had become very useless.

I turned to Lindsey and said, "Hey, I don't think this is right."

Lindsey was helping tug at the roots when she looked at my arm and yelled, "Christ Sarah, raise up your arm, get the hell out of the hole!"

I went and sat down on my front porch. It was late on a Sunday evening and after icing my arm for a while the swelling seemed to have gone down so I did not get it checked out. Looking back, I probably should have gone to the Emergency room right then and there. I decided to call the doctor the next day since the swelling came back. My surgeon ordered a Doppler test to look for a blood clot. A Doppler works the same as with the weather, except it is radar for your veins. The result was negative for a blood clot, so I went about my business. There was still soreness in my arm and the swelling never quite went all the way down. A couple of days later at work, it got worse. I called the doctor from work in-between meetings and was told to immediately go to the hospital for another Doppler test. This time they found a clot near my port. I was immediately admitted to the hospital, "Do not pass go and do not collect two hundred dollars." I started to freak out a little because I was by myself and the technicians were all talking like the clot could break loose at any moment and head for my brain. Fortunately, no stroke occurred and later that evening I was taken to surgery to have the port removed. I had called my aunt and also Lindsey to tell them where I was at and what was going on prior to the surgery. When I was wheeled back up to the room, I found my aunt, cousins, Lindsey and my friend Ginger all in the room taking turns wearing a wig. They were loud as shit and having a grand old time. They were in the middle of trying to get a nurse to try the wig on when I rolled up. The nurse was not amused. Lindsey had decided to buy me a wig and was testing it out on everyone. I was in another anesthetic haze so I was too fucked up to care. I was already pissed off that I had to stay the night in the hospital, which anyone who has stayed in one before, knows it involves getting your ass woken up every hour to get vitals taken. The next morning my surgeon came in and said I could go home in the afternoon, but she was going to put me on Lovenox and Coumadin, which are blood thinners. Lovenox involves giving yourself a shot in the stomach twice a day. Because my clotting level would never go to the correct level,—termed your INR number—I was forced to be on Lovenox for the duration of my chemotherapy. The shot caused spectacular bruising at the site of injection, and thus I looked like a domestic abuse victim from all the bruising.

Subsequently I was deemed the lumberjack at the oncologist's office. My oncologist scolded me for the tree stump incident, but in my defense I told him that he told me to do things that were normal when I felt like it.

He quickly responded, "Well I thought what was normal for me, I never thought that would include taking a hatchet to a tree stump."

Well, apparently normal for me is not normal to them. I tried to behave after that incident after I thought about the fact that I could have had a stroke. It turned out that I not only excelled at science, but at clotting as well.

After the port removal, I had to have a way to get my next dose of chemo. Because it was in a week, the doctors decided to put in a Peripherally Inserted Central Catheter line which is a catheter that is inserted in your inner bicep that runs all the way to your heart. Unlike the port, it hangs out and is a temporary solution. I went in for that procedure which was fairly quick and painless—no anesthetic, damn it. The line hanging out of my arm was very inconvenient and annoying—the cats were tempted to bat at it. I received my next dose of chemo and planned for another port. This time they were going to place it in my jugular since it was a wider vein, and less likely to clot. So I was off to surgery again for a new port. As I was awakening from anesthesia, I subconsciously knew that there was something wrong. My neck and chest was sore and I overheard them talking about the surgery not being successful. The surgeon tried to go into the original site in my chest and was unable to thread the port. She then tried to enter through one side of my neck and was again stonewalled. She subsequently tried on the other side of my neck and finally had to stop because I started bleeding. They decided to stop the surgery. Needless to say I was pissed, not at the surgeon, but at my fucked-up anatomy. Apparently my veins branch funky making threading the catheter difficult. I was the proud new owner of three scars and nothing to show for it. With the right do-rag, I looked like a biker chick who was in a serious knife fight. I was a hot commodity at the redneck bars.

The doctor sent me to Interventional Radiology (IR) to try to get the port in. This was now a day before I was scheduled to get my next dose of chemo. What IR does is surgically put the port in, but with the aid of X-ray and ultrasound. I was becoming a professional at minor surgery. In a sick way I started looking forward to the pleasant ride of post anesthetic bliss. The procedure was quick and I actually awoke while the doctor was still stitching up the site. Back in the recovery room, they stuck an external device into the port to test the return to make sure there were no clots. In a moment of sheer brilliance, the doctor decided to leave the external device plugged in since I was getting chemo the next day. I now had a big needle stuck in my IV port located under my skin on my chest. All this is wrapped on top with clear, new skin bandage over it to create pressure and stop any residual bleeding. Since I was still numb, I did not think twice about this set up. The doctor indicated that he was saving me from being stuck twice.

I went home to lie on the couch. As the anesthetic wore off, the pain started. Over the next few hours, the pain became unbearable. I normally have a high tolerance for pain and do not like taking prescribed pain killers because they tend to make me nauseous. So I rode it out until Lindsey came over to check on me. I wanted her to take the tape off as it was now so tight pressing on the needle stuck in my chest because what the genius doctor did not think about was that post operatively the area would swell. In addition, every time I moved my arm, the area would start to bleed. I was also still on blood thinners, not helping the situation. As she started to take the tape off, I apparently looked like I was about to pass out. She was able to get me patched up, but I was still bleeding. I also had discovered during all the surgeries that my skin was sensitive to the tape that was used to bandage me up, so she rigged a cornucopia of band aids and gauze, made me take Vicodin and laid my ass on the couch. I stayed there all night on my back because of the pain, bleeding with the external device still hanging out of my chest. By morning I had bled all over and was still in pain. But I had to suck it up because I was off to chemo.

At chemo, it took some convincing to get treatment due to the bleeding from where the needle was in the skin. Because the bleeding would not stop, after chemo, they sent me back to where I got the port put in to take a look at it and pull the external device out. After removing the device, they put pressure on the port area. It hurt like a mother fucker. They finally got it to stop bleeding; they bandaged the area and sent me on my way. As the evening progressed, every movement of my arm brought a fresh round of bleeding. If detectives would have gone through my trash, I would have been arrested for a suspected homicide. I could not get the area to stop bleeding, and to put pressure on the wound nearly caused me to pass out. Lindsey came over that night, as usual, to check up on me. When she saw my situation, she was beyond pissed. She called the IR department and the only person available was an on-call physician assistant (PA.)

She ended up bitching out this PA because she basically could not do too much about the problem and was referring us to an Emergency Room. Lindsey quickly countered that we were not going to have some new ER doctor, unfamiliar to the situation, begin to assess this problem when just grazing the surface of the skin where the port is located made me want to cringe in pain. She then told the PA that if she wanted us to put pressure and have me sleep with blood soaked clothes, then that was what we would do! Thankfully, after about another hour, the bleeding subsided enough that a bandage could absorb it. Lindsey, realizing that she had taken out her stress on the PA, did call her back to let her know that the bleeding had subsided and that we were going to make an appointment in the morning. The PA was glad that she had called back—probably thankful that it was a much calmer conversation.

The next day I was seen by the IR doc and ended up with a compression bandage which stopped the bleeding. In the end, I felt like the doctor did not make a very good pocket for the port under my skin. It stuck up so bad that even after the area healed it looked like the prongs of the port were coming through my skin. Because the skin was pulled so tight, the sutures would re-open with every movement of my arm. Every doctor that examined me afterwards commented on how bad it looked. I proceeded to suffer for the next eight weeks. Every time I moved wrong, including getting dressed, I was in pain.

On top of the port fiasco, I had just begun my new chemo drug: Taxol. While Taxol has no nausea associated with the treatment, the drug has its own special side effects. The possibilities are neuropathy (tingling or numbness in the hands and feet), arthralgia (joint pain) and turning of the fingernails and toenails brown, then falling off. Taxol also has a chromaphore in the formulation that many patients experience an allergic reaction to. Thus, you have to get a shitload of Benadryl before the actual Taxol, which is a three-hour infusion. You spend the first hour in a comatose state since Benadryl makes you very sleepy. The next two hours are spent trying to literally keep your ass from going numb in the recliner—and with no hot dudes there to massage it, you are left to shifting uncomfortably from side to side.

My luck was that I experienced the arthralgia. It felt like the growing pains that I had experienced as a child. The pain would last for about four days. On top of this joy, I still had to deal with the white blood cell booster shot to add to the party going on inside my blood stream. My week of chemo was spent either in the chemo lounge or on the couch in just enough pain to be miserable. By the end of the week, I could muster up enough energy to go to work and make others miserable. As I neared the end of chemo, I got progressively tired, but I also had a sense of excitement to get this shit over with and move on. On the day of my last chemo, I requested that the port get yanked out. So I suffered through my morning infusion with no liquids or food and moved to the surgical area and rode my MAC sedation cocktail to get my port removed. To celebrate, I slept on the couch all day and then went to a concert that evening. During chemo, I had become quite the cheap date, so my two drink maximum was met with authority.

I could now look forward to a few weeks off from torture. A few weeks off from doctor's appointments, blood draws and chemical infusions, and more importantly, normalcy in time to enjoy the Christmas holiday. If it was not for the bald head, I would have never have thought that I had gone through chemo, except for New Year's Eve where I pushed the drink limit and mixed my bourbons. New Year's Day found me back in my own familiar position—riding the couch with the kitties.

As I look back at my experience with chemo, I cannot even believe that I went through the process. It was certainly not what I expected. Chemo is doable if you listen to your body and communicate honestly with your doctor. Advances in anti nausea treatment and the ability to boost your immune system with new therapies like Neulasta allow the process to not be the horror show of the past. I will say it is not something that I ever want to go through again, mainly because of the disruption to your life more than feeling like shit. If you go into it with the right mindset from how to deal with your changing looks to how you will approach your treatment, you will be as prepared as you need to be to deal with the process with the right attitude. I believe if you go in there with a mindset that it will alter your life and you will get sick, then you will. Every time somebody tried to tell me how horrible it was to have to go through chemo, I ignored them. I wanted it to be my own experience. I cannot promise you that you will breeze through the treatment, but I can tell you to do everything possible to set yourself up for success.

Getting Wiggy With It

EXCERPT FROM AN EMAIL UPDATE, 8/28/2007:

"In 2 weeks, I will be Telly Savalas reincarnate. To prepare you all, I think you know that I am not a wig sort of girl, so I am going the do-rag route, so if you find any that are obnoxious and fit my personality, send them my way."

A big decision for chemo is what to do about the hair. Typically your hair falls out after the second treatment. I decided to cut my hair very short—it was already short, so not a big stretch—prior to starting chemo to not have a mess when it did fall out. During my initial visits to the chemo lounge I scoped out the different ways that people dealt with the hair loss. There was the do-rag contingent (my personal choice); the wrap (similar to the do-rag, but more formal looking—popular with the older ladies); the wig group and finally the ones that obviously had a hard time letting go so they wear nothing on their heads and have several bald patches with random strands of hair still attached. The last group I will never understand as it makes you look as bad as you feel.

After the second treatment of chemo, I got cocky as I still had my shiny mane and nothing was coming out. I thought just maybe I was that two percent that did not have hair loss. In fact I was actually fine with losing everything from the chin down. Two days after this thought, I was in the shower and as I was bathing, a clump of my nether region came out in the wash rag. Woo Hoo! No more having to wax and shave. Later that day, the hair on my head started coming out in clumps if I pulled on it. Emotionally, as well as hygienically, I did not want to spend my mornings waking up to large clumps of hair on my pillow. A phone call was made to my friends to inform them of this latest development. Lindsey decided that the shaving of the hair would occur that evening. Her step sister owned clippers so she came over to do the deed. I did not think it was a big deal until she started shaving. My resolve began to crumble because I realized that what I had been able to hide from the world would be painfully obvious. The world would look at me as a cancer patient, thus start giving me 'the look.' Thankfully. Lindsey being her usual self was cracking jokes throughout the whole thing.

"Demmon," she said, "you get five minutes and then we are going to move on."

So that is what I did. To make my statement to cancer and the world, I wore a Harley do-rag with skulls to work the next day, daring anyone to say shit to me. I knew that I had made the intended effect when a gentleman I did not know was walking out of a building as I was entering said, "Nice do-rag."

I put down the challenge to my friends to instead of shaving their heads to show solidarity—I would have never asked anyone to ruin their golden locks for me—that they should find creative do-rags to give me. I must have accumulated over fifty of them. I had ones for Halloween and Christmas, my sports teams, dressing nice or being sassy. I had let everyone know up front that I was not a wig sort of girl. Lindsey, however, decided I needed to have one just in case, so as I said before, she bought me one. I did have my cousin's wedding in the middle of chemo, so I was not totally opposed. I wore it to the wedding and also out one weekend. By the time my hair started growing back, I was sick of wearing anything on my head—the hot flashes did not help—so I went au natural. I had to get used to the staring again, but now people had choices as to my situation.

Was I devotee to the movie "GI Jane?" Was I an aging Goth chick? Was it the cancer?

I now had an air of mystery about me! All I can say is that what you do with your hair is a personal choice. Do what you feel comfortable doing. But please do not do the desperately hanging clumps. It looks like shit. Besides, your hair will grow back. Mine came back with a lot of gray. However, as it started to grow out, what I had heard came to fruition. My previously straight, fine hair came back wavy and thick. After about five months, however, the curliness wore off and I was back to straight hair. When it was long enough, I colored it red with blond flame tips. I wanted fire!

Reconstruction:
"How DIEP is Your Love?"

EXCERPT FROM EMAIL, 10/04/2007:

"I may have to wait 6 months to a year post mastectomy to get new girls."

For those of you getting lumpectomies, I have no advice for you, except for long term monitoring—get something better than a mammogram. Just the other day, a friend got a scare after her mammogram—you know, the nice phone call back saying that they found something, but will not give you a clue as to what they found, which side, etc. It turned out that the technician had accidentally double folded her skin causing a shadow. After my journey with missing the boat on a diagnosis, I am done relying on imagery, but I digress.

As I indicated, I went the double mastectomy route, even though as of now, the other side is healthy. I had no choice for the diseased side and as my friend said, "why keep saggy?" In reality, the choice to have a bilateral done was due to the inherent lumpiness in my breasts. Every lump I feel on the healthy side will keep me wondering, and I just do not want to live in fear of one of those lumps turning bad. Hey, I could write into Dr. Phil about my misbehaving lump—he could yell at it until it behaved. Maybe because I have not had kids or see that area as a huge pleasure zone—I would rather attention be focused in other areas, and as my friend Cindy said, "You can stay and chat, but let's not have a conversation."—it made the decision for me a no-brainer. It actually puzzles me when I read or hear about women who have so much attachment to what is now a diseased lump 'o' fat. If it was their pancreas, liver, kidney, etc., I think they would be less traumatized about getting those removed because you cannot see them, and those organs, while vital to your functioning, are not defining organs. The fact that your boobs are external, aesthetically pleasing to the opposite sex—or I guess the same sex if that is how you roll,—and are the quickest way to identify you as a woman, makes it hard to get rid of them. They are the center of nurturing for mothers and how you first bond with your child, and can make you feel sexy. But it is not like you are not getting a spare set, and hell, they may even be better than the first. I guess I just believe that sexiness and womanhood is a state of mind and so I made up my mind to getting new and improved models, working boobs if you will. I will be even sexier! And if I ever become a mother, natural or otherwise, there are other ways to form a bond with your child. In one of the books I was browsing through, the women spent an agonizing length of time saying good bye to her boobs the night before surgery. I said, "Good riddance to the bags of diseased fat!"

Well enough about the loss of the girls; let us talk about shopping for new ones. This is one area I really did not dig into like I should have in the beginning. As much effort that you put into deciding on your treatment, you need to put into your reconstruction options. Reconstruction means yet another doctor: the plastic surgeon. I have felt that this decision is the hardest, because of all the medical specialties, plastic surgery seems to be the diciest with respect to finding a surgeon that is reputable and good at what they do. I mean how many times do you hear about plastic surgery mishaps? Just watch the Discovery Health Channel one evening. I guarantee there will be a show on plastic surgery gone wrong. Make sure to ask around. I chose the first one I visited on the basis of word of mouth and the fact that my breast surgeon had worked frequently with this doctor, giving another level of comfort that there would be collaboration on the team. Make sure you ask to see pictures.

Some doctors post them on line, but do not look these up at work lest you get accused of looking at porn instead of working . . . Most should have a 'brag book' to show you in the office. Ask the doctor about their failures. By no means do you want to go into this without knowing all the risks associated with each procedure. Gauge the doctor's reaction to the failure question. Do they get defensive or do they express regret? Defensive is bad—expressing regret is better because they took the failure to heart and will hopefully try harder for you.

In the beginning, I had my mind set on implants. The only other choices I was aware of at the time involved cutting muscle and I was adamant about not losing my ability to be physically active at the same level as before all this happened. The way implants work is that they place a tissue expander under the chest muscle after the mastectomy surgery. A tube—one of several— runs externally where saline is gradually introduced to expand the surrounding tissue and skin until you reach the desired size. The expander is then removed and replaced with a permanent implant. If only one breast was removed, there will be some reconstruction on the other breast to make them match, if you desire. As far as from what I have read, nipple reconstruction with implants is not performed. A tattoo is done, again if desired, to recreate the areola and nipple, obviously with no texture. Or you can elect to go the Barbie route and do nothing. Again, a personal decision. The implant route means shorter recovery time—no muscle is cut—but the result looks the least natural . . . real working boobs—can you say Pamela Anderson! This seemed the choice for me until I was informed, and was subsequently confirmed by reading journal articles, that if you are going to have to do radiation, the success rate of implants is less than fifty percent. This is due to the damage to the skin that occurs during radiation. Plastic surgeons now refuse to even consider this option, even as a delayed reconstruction procedure for radiation patients. Yes I did say delayed. Before you get on the thought train that I did, do not think your journey is over at the mastectomy if you are to receive radiation. Most plastic surgeons will not reconstruct until six months to a year post treatment in order to let the area heal. This little nugget of information did catch me off guard and was the cause of a week of a shitty attitude.

So, back to my first visit to the plastic surgeon. I went to the appointment and clearly stated up front what I wanted my level of activity to be after the surgery. This immediately sent her into the most discouraging tone and pretty much in her body language I could tell that she had eliminated me as a potential patient. You see the other two choices are the TRAM flap and the latissimus flap. The TRAM flap involves cutting the muscle that runs the length of your stomach and folding it up to create the breast. It is then filled with fat from your belly—a tummy tuck to boot! This leaves you with only underlying rib muscle, and thus you will lose considerable strength. There is also the free TRAM where only a small section of the muscle is removed. In both cases, the chances of getting a hernia are very high—forty to sixty percent. I have also read some patient testimonials where they are unable to sit up without severe pain or help for several months, if not permanently. The latissimus flap involves cutting your entire lat muscle from your back and moving it to the front. In this case, you are only left with the underlying rib muscle as well. Common problems with this procedure are shoulder freezing, making lifting your arms above your head impossible and a decrease in strength—there goes my already shitty golf game—not to mention, disfigurement of your back.

The whole visit to the plastic surgeon was very bizarre. First, I was made to watch a video in a room, by myself, on reconstruction. She then came in to talk to me, or rather spread her blanket of negativity. What was worse is that she mentioned an alternative procedure not performed in Indiana, but did not offer any suggestions or recommendations on who was 'the bomb' in that area. She then proceeded to take pictures of my hooters in case I decided to become a patient—my first nude photos, Playboy, here I come—and sent me on my way. Needless to say, I left the office in a very foul mood.

The other procedure that she had mentioned is called the Deep Inferior Epigastric Perforator (DIEP) flap. This procedure is less invasive and does not involve the cutting of any muscle. Instead, the fat from your stomach, along with several blood vessels are moved up to create the breast. A tummy tuck and new hooters to boot! The biggest bonus is immediate recon-struction. No spending six months without boobs. The surgery is technically very difficult, thus the reason why not many doc-tors perform the procedure. Much to my ongoing good fortune, no one in Indiana performed the operation. Because the plastic surgeon I had seen was oh so helpful, I was left with my old friend the Internet to find myself a doctor. I typed in DIEP and let my search engines run wild. Through my surfing, I found the doctor who was credited as the pioneer of the procedure in New Orleans. Another hit intrigued me more, however. This was a doctor in New York. His website not only listed the fact that he had performed over eight hundred of the surgeries, but had testi-monials on how he was able to get insurance to pay for the pro-cedure. Of all the other websites discussing the procedure, this one interested me the most. I thought, "What the hell," and sent an email to the doctor. My friend suggested emailing Dr. Oz to ask him about the procedure. For all you non-Oprah fans, he is a charismatic doctor who appears once every couple of weeks or so on her show. I did so on the same night. Unfortunately, Dr. Oz never responded. Two nights later, Lindsey happened to be over at my house and at about 9:30 at night the phone rang. I started cussing because caller ID said it was unknown name and number which normally indicates a solicitor.

"What in the hell is a solicitor doing calling this late?"

My answering machine picked up and it was the doctor from New York. I was so shocked I think I stuttered for the first five minutes of the conversation. He was great on the phone. He explained the procedure to me in depth and how I would be the perfect candidate. What struck me about the doctor is that he openly talked about the fact that he had some failures is his career, but expressed deep regret about those failures and thought about them often. And unlike other doctors, instead of asking me about what I wanted to do, he told me what he thought I should do. The perfect combination: cockiness and sensitivity. To be cheesy, he had me at hello—oh yes; once in a while I am guilty of watching chick flicks. He gave me his office information and asked me to arrange a consultation. I called his office the first thing the next morning with a new feeling of hope. I made arrangements to fly out the following week to do a day in New York to meet the surgeon and hopefully find some answers. They also hooked me up with a breast surgeon in New York. You want the plastic surgeon and breast surgeon to be a team that knows each other and can work together. I should stop and explain here that the actual mastectomy is performed by the breast surgeon while the reconstruction is performed by the plastic surgeon.

I flew out the night before my appointment. Because of some bad weather, I did not get the flight until late. Let me preface this by saying that I have been to Europe several times, and even have been to New York City, but I am still proud to admit that I am a dumbass. Maybe it was because I did not have time to do my usual trip preparation of getting a car, printing out every view of Map Quest for all the places I was visiting and talking to local natives. I thought that for a one day trip, I would just cab it. When arriving in New York City, do not, I repeat, do not ever take a yellow cab from the airport to Long Island. I told the cabbie where I was going. "Sure, sure, I know where that is." He proceeded to accelerate on to the freeway with the pleasant stench of rotten curry in the air. Not more than five minutes into the cab ride, he asked where I was going again and then asked what exit to take.

I thought, "Oh shit I am screwed."

Fortunately I had prepared a little and had the hotel number with me. We pulled over—oh yes, the meter kept running—to call the hotel so that he could get directions. He then began cussing the guy out giving him directions for no apparent reason. However, he managed, or so I thought, to get the directions and so we headed off in the general direction. I was still slightly alarmed because he kept asking me the name and address of the place we were heading to. I began to imagine myself in the Amazing Race, trying desperately to communicate in another country—the country of New York—with an uncooperative cab driver. We pulled off to an exit that had at least the name of the city that I was going to and we passed by the hospital that the surgeon is associated with, which was another good sign. However, the cab driver had failed to acquire the final pieces of the directions, so we now had to stop at a gas station —oh yes, the meter was running, running, running, running—to get more directions. He found the final piece of the puzzle and we made it to the hotel where he dropped the next bombshell. The meter had one fee, but he did not explain the fact that by coming over to Long Island, there was an extra fee. The cab driver asked for $80. Gee, thanks for ass fucking me and then charging me for it. At that point, I just wanted to get out of the cab and into my bed. The asswipe did not even bother to get out and help me with my luggage. He popped the trunk and just sat there. Had I not been so tired, I would have thought quicker and walked off with the trunk open after retrieving my luggage.

My appointment was with the plastic surgeon first, followed by the breast surgeon at the end of the day, cutting close my flight home. The plastic surgeon's office was great. His staff was awesome. He has an insurance coordinator who works on convincing my insurance company that they would pay for me to go out of town to get this special procedure as opposed to the others that were available. When I met her, I knew it would not be a problem. She was a bulldog. She explained her whole game plan of how she would address every scenario that the insurance company might come up with. Let me stop the bus a minute to explain that by law, insurance must pay for reconstruction. However, they do not have to pay for what you choose. An important lesson to be learned is that if you have to go 'out of network' to get the surgeon or procedure you want, fight the insurance company. Meet with your surgeon's insurance coordinator to come up with a game plan to get what you want, not what insurance wants. You have been through enough shit; you should get what you deserve.

After meeting with the doctor, I knew right then and there that was what I wanted. He showed me his brag book which consisted of before and after pictures. Let me tell you, he does a great work. He had dealt with many shapes and sizes and also fixed situations where other plastic surgeons had screwed up. I was very impressed, to say the least. I committed to a down payment when I said yes. You are not allowed to say yes for seven days—do not ask me why. I am not sure that a down payment is the norm with plastic surgeons, since they have different services which are not covered by insurance. I just know that this is what I had to do to commit to this doctor. The down payment of almost $10,000 was submitted to insurance, but I did not recoup the amount until after the surgery, when the claim was filed.

I also met with the general surgeon when I was there. She also was great and I felt very much at ease with her. I am of the mindset of not caring if my doctor has a total asshole personality, just as long as they are competent. It is a bonus to me if we mesh. I can say that during this whole ordeal, I was lucky to have ended up with doctors that suited me very well.

Within a week of getting back to Indianapolis, I called the plastic surgeon and said, "Yes!"

They gave me a date for surgery and began the process of negotiating with the insurance company. I informed all my doctors of my decision. They were all very supportive. Fortunately, my breast surgeon in Indy knew of someone who had gotten DIEP done and was whole-heartedly on board. She offered to do all my follow up and to help me find a plastic surgeon in Indy to finish the easy part of the reconstruction, the nipple and areole, if I did not want to go back out to New York.

I started making arrangements for my trip. I needed to be in New York for a total of ten days. Three days would be in the hospital and the rest recovering at a hotel. Lindsey immediately said she would go. My aunt also wanted to go as well as my mom. I had no idea of what I was going to need other than the little bit of information given to me by the doctor. My selection of hotel was based purely on the internet and location near the doctor. I wanted one that was like an efficiency that people stay in for extended business trips as I did not want to be cooped up in one room all day and I did not want to eat junk all week. In retrospect, I should have talked to the doctor's office in New York sooner about my arrangements, but it all worked out in the end. My independence in doing things almost bit me in the ass, though.

Surgery—
Not For the Faint of Heart

EMAIL EXCERPT, 2/11/2008:

"I was in the worst pain in my life. I was okay if I died that day because I was sincerely miserable. For any of you considering a tummy tuck, think twice."

As the new year dawned, I had a month to prepare for surgery both mentally and at work. My hair was growing back, so I had ditched the do-rags, which resulted in everybody and their mother petting my head as they talked to me. My love of my personal space being invaded was sorely tested.

During this time, one of my kitties died. The radiation oncologist was insisting on radiation before even seeing the outcome of surgery and work was back to the norm of fifty hours a week. So much for mental preparation, more like mental survival. I had made all my arrangements—or so I thought—for myself and my traveling entourage. For the first week, my mom and uncle were going to be with me. They would then leave and my aunt, cousin and Lindsey would come out for the second week while I was convalescing at the hotel.

I was wanting the days to fly by so that I could get surgery over with. It did not help that people were being supportive with comments such as "Are you scared?" or "Are you nervous?"

"No, but thanks for bringing it up."

No matter what my state was, it was not like I had a choice. Well I take that back. I had the choice of not having the surgery and dying of cancer eventually, I guess. A week before surgery, I had to get all these pre-surgery tests done—blood work, chest x-ray, etc. I called the doctor in New York to let them know that they should be expecting these results and off handedly mentioned my choice of hotel. The doctor's office indicated they would check out the facility and call me back. Well not five minutes later, I got a phone call.

"Oh honey, you have to get out of that hotel. They busted prostitutes there last week".

So much for my internet savvy to select a hotel that rents rooms by the hour—although I could have worked off some of my financial debt…. The doctor's office promised to look into alternatives for me. I started to really stress out as I was supposed to leave in six days. They called me back the following day to tell me they had found an alternative: a senior assisted living facility.

I thought, "A nursing home? You have got to be kidding me."

But then they described the facility. It consisted of small apartments with on-site nursing, meals and a driver. Seeing that I had little choice at this point, I accepted the arrangement. I went on the net and checked out the website and it actually did not look too bad. They showed happy old people smiling and playing Wii®.

I thought, "Hey, I could get into some Bingo."

The weekend before I left, I had one last hurrah with my friends. I behaved myself as I did not think a hangover would have been good for traveling and surgery. I started packing the day before my flight and just threw a bunch of shit into the suitcases. I had delusions of grandeur that I would be running around New York City the second week, so I packed jeans and shirts for those situations, pajama pants for lying around and shorts and t-shirts for working out. Let me tell you what you really need: pajama pants and loose shirts. You will also want to get the Hanes™ undershirts—that are known affectionately as wife beaters—as they help with containing all the apparatus that you will have on when you come home from the hospital. You will not be wearing jeans anytime soon after surgery. You will not be working out and you will not be running around any city.

My mom met me in Indianapolis for the flight out. She was in a wheel chair due to foot problems, so I had to wheel her and all the bags through the airport, but I did it gladly out of love…. We arrived at the senior facility in the morning. I had doctors' appointments later in the afternoon, so I wanted to get settled. The place was great and could not be more perfect. In fact because of me, the doctor decided to recommend all their out of town patients from then on to stay there. The rooms were small, but hey, that is New York. They had a shower with a seat, which you need the first week when you come home from the hospital, a med alert bracelet to call the staff 24-7 if you needed anything. They provided meals if we wanted them and a driver to take us to different appointments. The entire staff was very helpful and the residents were a trip. My family thoroughly enjoyed staying there. When my mother and I first showed up, I had to laugh because they thought I was moving her in. I do not think she found it very funny. In fact I think my family was a little worried that I may have had an ulterior motive in selecting the place in case I was looking for a permanent residence for them. The first time we went into the room, the heat was blasting. I ran the air conditioning the entire two weeks as the temperature in the building was set for old people with no circulation, not young people with hot flashes.

We went to see the breast surgeon and the plastic surgeon that afternoon. The plastic surgeon spent about an hour drawing all over my chest and stomach and using Doppler to identify viable blood vessels. He then explained the most important thing you need to also know before surgery: There is always a chance that the surgeon will get in there and find out due to a whole host of reasons that he cannot conduct the reconstruction at that time. So you need to be prepared for a small chance that you could wake up and not be reconstructed. This does not mean that reconstruction can never be done. It just means you will have to wait.

I was not allowed to shower that night. Mom and I capped off the evening by eating dinner. Choose wisely because this meal will stay with you literally for a week, so my recommendation is to select a light meal. My uncle flew in later that night. At 5am the next morning, I headed for the hospital. My surgery was to be at 7:30 in the morning and I can honestly say I was not nervous or scared. I just wanted to get over it. As the magic hour approached, I was walked into the operating room for my date with destiny. I remember hopping up on the table, asking for a pillow for under my knees and began to feel the warm fuzzy feeling of going down the anesthesia highway. While I am sure it was a long day for my family, it was the shortest day of my life. The breast surgeon was the first on the stage with the mastectomy and the sentinel node biopsy. She came out around noon to let my family know that her portion was complete. The nodes were negative and there appeared to be no involvement of the tumor with the chest wall. Both facts were excellent pieces of news.

My reconstruction surgery ended up lasting until 11pm. I just know I went to sleep in a warm fuzzy cocoon and woke up in sheer hell. Immediately upon waking, I was nauseated and began throwing up. Thank God I was still numb because that would have hurt like hell. I remember briefly my mom and uncle coming in, and then going back to sleep. They hooked me up to morphine which I could self medicate with every six minutes. That next day I wanted to die. I will not sugar coat it, I felt like I had been hit by a truck.

I remember lying there and thinking "what have I done?" My throat was on fire from being intubated for sixteen hours, but I could not drink because of the nausea. Finally, a nurse began feeding me ice chips. Those nuggets of ice tasted better than any beer that I had ever had. Later that afternoon they moved me to a room. Because I was in a large bed, they had to crank me up into a sitting position to get me into the elevator. The assistants started bitching about the bed size, the amount of extraneous equipment that came with me and the standard of care that I was getting versus others. I thought for sure they were going to dump me somewhere—paranoid on pain medication, there is nothing better. They did not realize that the doctor had placed extra sensors on me to monitor the oxygenation of my skin to make sure everything he did took. The ride up to my room was pure hell. I became motion sick and was in excruciating pain. I began to realize that I was not in a nice Midwestern hospital where everyone is cordial and the rooms are roomy and cozy. The hospital was huge, the rooms were small and the people were in a hurry. I was told if I wanted to watch T.V., I had to pay for it.

"What the Fuck? I have to be in this tiny room for how many days, I can't sit up to read and you are not going to provide T.V.? Gee, I think I will pay."

The nurses told me that I would be getting out of bed that evening into a chair. Logic and advice from others told me that mobility was the key to getting better. However, pain and nausea were telling me that there was no way in hell that I was moving from that position for the rest of my life. I ate some pineapple and continued my prayer for a swift ending to my suffering. As the day wore on, I became conscious of my body and what was done to it. I had a catheter plus eight drains hanging out of me— two under each armpit and four coming out of just below my bikini line. These drains were almost as thick as drinking straws ending in 50mL bulbs and were stitched into my skin with thick, black thread. They had to be milked of fluid every few hours which involved the nurse pulling on the drains. I quickly learned to take a hit of morphine before they came in because it hurt like hell when they pulled on them. I could not see the end result of the surgery yet: my new boobs. All that I knew at the time was that everyone said they looked good. The nurses and doctors continually checked the capillary refill on the breast by pushing on it and looking to see if the blood returned. They were totally numb, so I did not feel anything for that test—one of the few.

The time had come that evening to sit up. The nurse slowly helped me to a sitting position on the bed. This took about 5 minutes as every motion caused an enormous amount of pain. After achieving the sitting position, they then stood me up and slid me into a chair. Several things occurred at this point. I started getting nauseous from the exertion and began a round of vomiting that was so painful that in between bouts, I swore like a sailor. After about five minutes of sitting, the oxygen sensors starting alarming so they put me back into bed. I was more than happy to go back to my reclining position. I took a hit on the pain pump and promptly drifted off into a happy haze. That evening, the fire in my back started from lying in an uncomfortable hospital bed in the same position. I laid there and wondered how others dealt with this. I mean there are some people that get their entire chest cracked open for heart surgery, and a lot of them are not young. Or was I wimpier than I thought I was? I was not lying in bed groaning or complaining, but I was not a ray of sunshine either.

The next morning, a new wrinkle was introduced. They removed the catheter which now required me to get up every couple of hours to pee. I had to page the nurse every time I needed to go because I could not get out of bed by myself. I felt totally helpless. And in true hospital fashion, the nurse could not always come when paged.

The doctor came in later that evening and informed me of two facts. One was that they were taking away the morphine— I was very sad— but giving me Percocet, which I only got a couple of doses before they took those away too—damn.

The other fact was posed as a question "Have you gotten out of bed by yourself yet?"

"No," I answered.

I took that question as a challenge to get my ass out of bed. I waited until about 2am when no one was around. I did not want my mom telling me to take it easy and I wanted to do it in my own way. It took me a while, but I achieved an exit from my prison bed and went to the restroom by myself. If I had not been so miserable, I would have done a victory dance. Friday morning, day three in the hospital, the doctor came in and I proudly informed him of my walking achievement. I expected a gold star! I got something better: a ticket out of jail. I was to be discharged that afternoon and sent to my temporary residence in the senior assisted living facility. Mind you, I still had my drain necklace as they were pinned to a strand of gauze around my neck which I had to keep on for at least a week or until they produced less than ten milliliters total of fluid in twenty-four hours.

That afternoon, my mom and uncle showed up to escort me out of the hospital. As everyone was preoccupied with getting me into the car, no one noticed that my stubborn mother had elected to roll herself in her wheelchair to the car instead of waiting for help. I did not witness this first hand, thankfully, for I would have busted my stitches open laughing, but she lost control on a slight down slope and rolled into traffic, which thankfully was stopped. She ended up with tire burn on her fingers from trying to brake the wheelchair. My uncle went to retrieve her as I painfully slid into the vehicle to freedom. The ride back was a test of car sickness and pain for every pothole that the driver hit caused a searing pain in my abdomen. When we arrived, I insisted on walking to my room. I can say it was the longest one hundred yards of my life.

The first thing when I got to my room was take off my clothes and check out my new look for the first time. I had not been able to see anything in the hospital, so this was my first time looking at the new me. To be honest, it was not as freaky as I thought it would be to look at boobs with no nipples. I had seen pictures, but it is different when it is you. I was pleasantly surprised as to how nice they looked. I had heard the comments from others, but seeing is believing. The only thing that was really disturbing to look at was the hoses coming out of my body. They looked as painful as they felt!

The next thing I did was shower. Now the amazing thing was I had no bandages anywhere on my body. All I had was my lovely gauze necklace of drains, yet I had been told I could shower. The beautiful thing about the senior assisted living facility was that the shower had a seat in it, which I needed. Lifting your hands easily above your head will not be a feat that you will be able to accomplish until several weeks out from surgery, so by sitting, it facilitated showering with no assistance. After my shower, I removed the gauze and replaced it with a ribbon necklace that had been provided by the doctor's office to re-pin the drains. The necklace was part of a goody bag full of all sorts of useful things. The goody bag had been donated by an organization called 'Necessities bag.' They had also provided these little pillows you can hold under your arms—they helped for sleeping—wound care products and a pad of paper to record your drain output. Yes, I did say drain output. You see, when you go home, your drains still need emptying. I believe the normal procedure is to have a home nurse come in and do this for you. I opted out of having someone come in because my cousin was coming that evening and was a registered nurse. I figured she could do the task and earn her room and board! In true geek fashion, I decided to chart my drain output in an Excel® graph so that I could monitor which drains were getting to a low output. I subsequently emailed the results to my doctor the night before seeing him. He was amused, to say the least.

Later that evening, the next shift of caregivers arrived: my aunt and cousin. My mom and uncle were to leave the next morning. I happily drifted off in a Vicodin haze as they went out for dinner and drinks. There was concern on my mother's part on who would be sober enough to wheel her back home. The rest of the family solicited the bar owner in case they were above the legal limit for drinking, walking and wheeling. Needless to say they all made it back fine. The next morning, the first shift of family left and I settled into what would be my routine for the next few days. This routine involved showering—for what I needed help getting undressed, drying off and dressing—then, watching TV interspersed with either reading or napping. My appetite was still pretty much nothing. I tried to be good and drink water all day with only a couple of Diet Pepsi's. My water intake was maybe three to four bottles a day, which in hindsight was not enough. We will get to why in a moment. My other form of self torture was to not take anything but Motrin during the day, saving the Vicodin for night time. My rationale around taking pain killers is as follows: First, I hate Vicodin. It hurts my stomach, making me very nauseous. Second, it gives me very violent dreams. Third, I believe that the more pain I could tolerate, the faster I would get better. No pain, no gain, right?

I had no choice but to take the Vicodin at night because I could only lie in one position which was on my back. The only way I could fall asleep was to take the pill.

After two days of this routine, the dynamic was about to change as Lindsey arrived in town. She knocked on the door and asked in the spirit of Tommy Boy, "You wan' pillow?"

She stayed in the room with me, so I now had jackass to deal with. Actually, it was a welcome sight as I had been without my peeps for over a week and needed the entertainment. Although, the bad thing about Lindsey and I staying in the same room on any trip is that every evening, what innocently starts as the intention to go to bed turns into anywhere from a half hour to an hour of sheer foolishness. She claims that I start it; I completely blame her. It will be quiet and all of the sudden a comment is made. This comment then leads to a whole slew of comments of which neither of us will stop. The problem with this foolishness is that it hurt me like hell to laugh, so this was going to be an exercise on my restraint to not start or join into any post lights out conversation.

When she arrived, I was finishing my post shower routine of milking my drains. I had fired my cousin after the first time she had tried because she was not performing the task to my satisfaction. I also hated anyone else touching the drains as it pulled on the stitched area and hurt.

I walked out into the living area with my drain necklace and said, "You might as well check it out."

I figured I might as well start off the visit with my alien drains and new boobs as nothing was going to be sacred with respect to my body by the end of the trip. In fact, I now have no trouble flashing anyone. I am ready for Mardi Gras. My new boobs are so much prettier than the older models that I cannot help myself.

Lindsey made some smart ass comment to which I made my usual reply, "Don't worry, in a week you will be wiping my ass."

"I am going to come over there and kick your ass, drains and all," I said.

She replied, "What? Are you going to beat me with your ninja drains?"

As she was saying this, she was swinging her arms about wildly as if having nunchuks in her hands. This became the running joke throughout the rest of the time I had the drains. I would pretend to swing them about wildly—actually doing this would have caused me to pass out in severe pain—in preparation for attack. Any bystander would think the two of us were twelve years old. This is what I mean by sheer foolishness.

During my time lounging about the room, I only went out once a day for a brief walk. I thus became the big mystery of the senior assisted living community. No one ever saw me. They saw people going in and out of the room, but never the guest of honor. Imagine a true New York accent saying, "How's your friend? Is she doing all right? We haven't seen her?"

However, my family was a different matter. They interacted with everyone and were in on all the dirt. They would come back to my room each night with new tidbits of information. One resident was having Asian call girls come to his apartment twice a week. Another turned 102 and they were going to get a card for her. The volunteer driver was taken with my mom and when she was gone, kept asking me how she was. I found their involvement with the residents absolutely hilarious. I was glad they were enjoying their time and could find other things to occupy their mind besides me. And of course they were all working on their New York accents, which is a far cry from the Hoosier twang. In retrospect, I could not have asked for a nicer place to stay.

My fifth day there, I was eating a little more, but another problem was beginning to rear its ugly head. I had not had a bowel movement since before surgery, which was now over a week ago. This is common post surgery. I had my caretakers go out and get me stool softeners to try to move the process along, but to no avail. That morning, I ate breakfast and soon after became very dizzy. I was so dizzy I thought I was going down. Lindsey said, "Demmon, today you will be taking a dump."

I had to have her help me get to the bathroom for fear of passing out. I could not go. They went out and got me some magnesium citrate. The stuff was so horrible to drink, but worked its magic within ten minutes of choking it down. I felt like I had shit out a bowling ball. I was able to thankfully wipe my own ass, which was about the only shred of dignity that I had left. I shuffled out of the bathroom, but immediately became faint and had to lie down. The vertigo was still there whenever I tried to raise my head. Lindsey made the executive decision to call the doctor. The doctor was concerned that my blood level may be low and I might need a blood transfusion, so he wanted me to go to the emergency room to have blood drawn as he could get results quicker than if I went to his office. The facility lent us a wheel chair and the driver. We then left for the hospital. We registered and then did not wait long to go back to the triage area. I naively thought that this would be an easy trip getting in so quickly. Boy was I wrong. After taking my vitals, we were placed in a holding area. I was whisked away for an electrocardiogram. The nurse administering the test began asking all sorts of questions about my plastic surgeon and the job he did that I felt obligated to flash her too. After complementing my rack, she tested me and sent me back to the holding area, which was right by the doors to where the ambulances brought in patients. It was about thirty degrees outside, so every time doors opened, everyone froze. We procecded to wait there forever. During the wait, they would bring in patients from the ambulance that were, for the most part, elderly. One man with gangrene and a bleeding ulcer in his foot was placed right in front of our chairs. I thought my aunt was going to throw up. Two hours into sitting in the waiting room, my doctor showed up to try to expedite me through. I think I might still be sitting there to this day if he had not intervened. I learned that even though Indianapolis is a big city with big hospitals, the city will never experience the volume of patients that a New York hospital will. The emergency room alone had seventy beds. Hell, we have hospitals in Indy that do not have that many beds in the whole place.

We were eventually moved to another area. The general consensus was that I was dehydrated. Even though I thought I was drinking enough, between losing fluid to the drains and being in the hole already from my hospital stay, I apparently was not getting enough fluids. My advice in retrospect is that as soon as you can, drink a shitload of water. After getting two liters of fluid, I felt tons better and we headed for home. This was a four-mile drive. Now the problem was that the senior facility driver was off by this point—five hours after we went to the hospital—so we had to call a cab. The problem was compounded by the area getting what they called their first significant snow fall of the season—a whole inch of snow. Coming from Indiana where you can get six inches in a drop of a hat, it was a mystery to all of us what the big deal was. It took us over an hour to go those four miles. I was in hell yet again. Could nothing be easy?

Two days after my emergency room visit, the time came to follow up with the doctor. I was hoping to get my drains out as we were to leave the next day for Indy. I knew that if I could just get them out, I would feel tons better. By this time, the entry points were very red and raw from moving around. They were my biggest source of discomfort and lack of sleep. I went into the office with the realistic view that I could very well be flying back with the things in. As soon as I showed the physician's assistant my drain output numbers, she stated that they were all coming out. I was ecstatic. My euphoria soon faded as she began the procedure of removing them. There was no numbing or preparation. She just began to cut all my stitches out and pulled the drains. I will not lie. It was a tad bit painful.

Lindsey kept yelling at me, "You better breathe Demmon," but the discomfort was inhibiting the process. I did manage to flip Lindsey off, however. The whole time I just focused on the fact that they were coming out, not on the pain. Soon she was done. I got my marching orders from the doctor. I was to come back in four to six months—depending on if I got radiation or not—to complete the reconstruction (nipples and areola.) As I put it, to get the icing on the cake. I was free to go home. I could not contain my excitement. Returning home and healing meant another step to becoming a normal, cancer-free human being.

In the running course of my luck, the trip back was anything but smooth. My aunt, in concern over getting me bumped by anyone and in her desire to press our advantage, an invalid, insisted on getting a wheel chair when we got to the airport. At this point, I could walk, albeit slowly, but could not carry more than my purse. By getting the wheel chair, we got to run right to the front of the security line. However, this meant that my wheel chair bound ass was placed at the point where you put your shoes back on to get frisked by security in front of God and everyone.

The female security guard started to press on my chest and stomach to which I had to say, "Hey, wait a minute, I just had surgery there, please do not press on that area." I think I might have ended up in a prison cell if she would not have listened because my reflex would have been to bitch slap her.

They then wheeled me to the gate. The gate agent immediately saw us and asked if we needed assistance for the flight. Now that she had saw my predicament, this meant that I needed to be wheeled everywhere in the airport, including the bathroom. Lindsey was laughing at me on the inside as she saw my face of sheer pissiness. I am not one to draw attention to myself, which being in the wheel chair automatically did. This also meant I wheeled in front of everyone to get on the plane. The passengers on the plane must have thought a miracle occurred mid flight, however, as I refused a wheel chair when we got to Indy and promptly walked to the baggage claim area. Lindsey's husband picked us up and took me home. I was never so glad to see my house as I was that day. I then realized how much shit I store above my head. At this point I could not lift my arms above my head and was under a weight restriction of lifting up no more than ten pounds. Try going to the grocery store and coming home with bags that weigh less than that. You do not realize how much you use certain muscles or your arms in general, for that matter.

The Road to Recovery

IN MY FINE TRADITION of not doing anything I should, the first evening home I put together a little file cabinet for Lindsey's daughter.

Lindsey's husband relayed this to another friend after being asked how I was doing. He said, "True to form she is not behaving as instructed. I could just see the potential of all the internal stitches starting to go pop, pop, pop, followed by two big globs of fat falling on the floor after assembly of the final shelf. The stuff is after all just sewn on."

Fortunately nothing like this occurred. Lindsey dragged my ass to the mall for a three-hour excursion the following day. I bought my first bras for the new me. The day was then topped off with a family get together at Lindsey's cousin's house—I am a surrogate member of the family. Towards the end of the evening, I was pretty much done. I never knew such little activity could be so exhausting.

I visited work to take care of some banking and became aware of a whole new way of getting the look. It was no longer the pity look. It was the stare and talk at my boobs for ten minutes before actually talking to my face. I was very amused as I could understand that if you knew someone was getting new hooters, the natural inclination would be to check them out. Besides, I thought they were pretty. In fact, I had started acting like a party goer at Mardi Gras, except that I would show them for free, though not at work, of course. Not one bead would need to be thrown at me.

It just became too lengthy to try to explain what they looked like so I would be like, "Here, I will just show you."

I did not flash guys, if that is what you were thinking, however. I did have some limits to my exhibitionism. And while I had gotten used to the no-nipple look, and I knew that my fellow females would be okay with it, I was not ready for gentlemen's scrutiny. I began to actually wonder if I hooked up with some guy before completion of the work, how would I prepare him for what he may see.

I began to think of fun scenarios: "My nipples were ripped off in a freak laboratory accident. See that box on the mantle—I keep them in there;" or "I sent them out to be cleaned;" or "My friend is wearing them, they go better with the outfit she has on."

Being that none of that happened, I have no advice as to date as to how you deal with the boyfriend, spouse or significant other post mastectomy. If you did not have immediate reconstruction, I can only imagine how hard psychologically it is for some. I know that when I thought that I was going to have to wait for six months before getting reconstruction, I was not happy. I knew that I would want a prosthesis and was thinking more of the pain in the ass it would be to deal with that during the summer. I could imagine driving a golf shot and one of them flying off the tee with the golf ball. This also meant no swimming, not that I am a big pool person, but enjoy it once in a while. I can say that not having nipples did not give me pause or cause me any emotional trauma. I go back to your inner core and self confidence in how you define yourself whether this would be a problem.

The first week that I was back from New York, I had an appointment with the radiation oncologist to discuss my pathology results. Before I left for surgery, the radiation oncologist was pretty insistent on my having radiation. However, I had seen my local breast surgeon a couple of days before and she was of the opinion that I did not need radiation. My post-surgery pathology report was stellar: no lymph node involvement; final size of the tumor was 1.5 cm; no chest wall involvement and the other breast was negative. I was glad I made the decision to have the other breast taken off as the report indicated that it was eighty percent fibrous. I would never have been able to tell a lump from fibrous tissue and would be thinking for the rest of my life that there were tumors in there.

The only reason that radiation was proposed in the first place was due to the hand measurement taken by my oncologist. There were several measurements taken of the original tumor before chemo. The tumor was measured by MRI, ultrasound and by hand. The oncologist measured 5.5 cm by hand and even stated that he tended to overestimate the size. The measurement by MRI was 3.5 cm, however. The cutoff for size for radiation is 5 cm. My hesitation at radiation was the fact that it was every weekday for six weeks. The main side effect was an increasing tiredness. More importantly, there was a good risk of encapsulation of the skin and my new pretty boobs would not be so pretty anymore. My good friend's sister had radiation and had also told me about sores that would not heal for months.

I went to my appointment ready to accept my fate. As the radiation oncologist started laying out the scenarios for treatment, I brought up the fact that the hand measurement was different from the MRI measurement, which was smaller than the standard size believed to have benefit versus risk for radiation. He had not even looked at the MRI number and was solely going on the hand measurement from the oncologist. This goes to show that you really need to read all your medical charts and reports as there may be details that are glossed over by any of the physicians that you deal with. If you cannot understand the basics of the report, find someone that can help you out. This doctor had just seen the hand measurement and made up his mind. He began to lay out the argument of accuracy of measurement between the different techniques and after keeping me on a hook for a good ten minutes indicated that MRI was probably the most accurate of all the measurements and thus, he agreed that no radiation was necessary. I could not believe it. I wanted to skip down the hall of the hospital. I was absolutely elated.

My elation was somewhat dampened the following week when I went to the oncologist for my first meeting with him as a cancer free individual. I knew that we would be discussing the next phase of treatment, but I had not really put a lot of thought into that visit. He was genuinely pleased with the outcome of my surgery and more importantly the final pathology report. The conversation soon segued into what was next. For estrogen positive tumors, chemo is really a secondary treatment. The primary treatment is estrogen modulation/suppression therapy. The standard of treatment has been Tamoxifen. Tamoxifen basically works by competing with estrogen for binding of the estrogen receptor. While this has been the standard treatment, I had hesitation from the first time I read about the drug with respect to taking it. The side effects are a risk for uterine and endometrial cancers, and blood clots. Because of my impressive history with clots, if I were to take Tamoxifen, I would need to be on a blood thinner for five years. Taking the risk of acquiring a different cancer was not an appealing option to me, since I was young and had plenty of time to incubate more tumors. Newer therapies involve aromatase inhibitors. These, however, are only prescribed in post-menopausal women because the primary mechanism of these drugs is to inhibit estrogen production by attacking their hormonal precursor. In post-menopausal women, estrogen production is low, making the drug more effective. For pre-menopausal women, the only way for the drug to work is to put the individual into menopause by irradiating the ovaries, removing them or receiving a shot in the ass on a routine basis that places you into menopause and then maintains that state. Of course, menopause means also means the joy of hot flashes. As my oncologist began to explain the various choices, it very slowly dawned on me that he was asking me to make a life choice. If I was going to choose what was behind door number one, I was to spend five years taking a drug that may or may not cause another type of cancer along with blood thinners that would mean injecting myself again once a day causing severe bruising in my ass—there was no way I was going to mess up my stomach again after the surgery—and/or random bruises that would show up by just bumping into things. Door number two meant the conscious choice that I would not have children natu-rally, because I was not going to wait until the age of forty-three to have children—there is too much risk to both the child and to myself. The big risk with aromatase inhibitors is the chance of loss of bone density due to the stoppage of estrogen production and random joint pain.

I sat there for a minute thinking, "Wow, I have to make a life decision within the next five minutes."

Some persuasion was offered by the oncologist who said if it was him in this situation, he would choose the aromatase inhibitor. It was a hard decision to make, but I choose the aromatase inhibitor route. I guess I knew deep down when the cancer journey started that the possibility of a child of my own was going to be remote, but I just was not prepared that day to pull the trigger. The whirlwind of activities that had gone on during my diagnosis left no time to think of my fertility. Maybe if someone would have sat down with me during that time and explained what would happen on the back end of all this, I may have taken pause on the subject of my eggs. However, considering my state of mind in wondering about the cancer, I probably still would not have explored the option of harvesting eggs as my brain was not working right. Thus, it was very much a kick in the gut for me to make the decision to go the menopause route, but I just felt that I wanted to go with the more current treatment and that the risks for the one medication were less than the other. I guess I should wait ten to twenty years to publish this book to let you know which door held the better prize package.

Four weeks out from surgery as I was making my rounds of doctors' appointments, I began to test my physical strength. I went to the gym and jogged one and a half miles and walked half a mile. Since my chest was absolutely numb, it did not bother me to run. My stomach, however, was another matter. The skin was pulled so tight that it was very difficult to take a deep breath. My ability to work out was a testament to the superiority of the surgery. I do not think that anyone having muscle cut could have done the same. Then the siren song of work began. The workaholic in me could not help it. First of all, there is not shit on TV during the day. I had already gotten several high scores on the Wii®. My brain felt like it was slowly rotting. I made the decision to go back to work the following week. Physically, I was getting better every day. The only hesitation about going to work was that I would get very sore in my stomach area when sitting for long periods of time. I had to make sure that I got up out of my chair periodically. In the grand tradition of the practical jokes that I so often play on others, my entire cube was decorated with pictures of owls. Usually my mind is in the gutter, but for some reason I did not get it right away. After asking one of my co-workers, the light bulb went on. It was a way to welcome my new hooters! The first couple of days back were spent recounting my surgery, but routine soon took over and normalcy began to assert itself again.

A Return to Society

EMAIL EXCERPT, 1/28/2008:

"The first day I tried to run, I could only go about a mile and was thoroughly pissed off until I had to remind myself that I had just gone through 4 months of chemo."

My body felt the fire of a thousand suns. Yet another hot flash. Two months after the surgery, life was slowly returning to normal. Physically, I was getting stronger. I was running a couple of days a week. My goal was to run the Race for the Cure which was just two months after surgery. Running was made tough because when I started to breathe hard, I couldn't recover because my stomach was so tight from the incision. I would get frustrated until I reminded myself that most people that had a double mastectomy with reconstruction would not be insane enough to be out running right after the surgery. Exercise, though was a must for me. I was getting full into work again which meant stress. I was also not sleeping very well because I woke up all the time with the hot flashes. To add insult to injury, the hormonal battle in my body was making me angry and my patience was very thin. I found myself battling with how to return to my place in life. For the past eight months, my world was focused on cancer. I was struggling with how to divert that focus back into the normal hustle and bustle of life.

The attention on my body from others was also an adjustment. Men had typically addressed my boobs in conversation before, but now everyone was talking to them. I got questions from everyone. I enjoyed the shock value of pointing out I had no nipples, which many did not realize. One day at work, one of my coworkers was excited about getting a back ordered shipment and was dancing around the lab. I could not help myself, so I said, "If I had nipples, I would be excited." I think the other two guys in the lab may have wet their pants in laughter.

I felt that I was in a kind of limbo, since I still had a couple of more surgeries to go. One surgery was to fix my sides and the final surgery was getting my nipple reconstruction. The incision that ran across my belly ended mid way on my sides. The effect was termed 'dog ears' in that there were two large puckers on either side. Not only was this irritating with clothing, but not very attractive as well. My breast surgeon had a plan to extend the incision around to my back on either side. This would again put me out of physical activity for yet another period of time. The weather was getting warm which meant the start to golf, softball and yard work. My impatience to complete my physical transformation outweighed my desire to take a reprieve from more physical torture.

My first goal, however, was the Race for the Cure. Lindsey and I had starting running the race about ten years before because her aunt had breast cancer. We had also used the race as a speed workout before running the Mini Marathon. In the past, I had shown up, run the race and headed home, usually then straight to the ball field for opening day for Lindsey's sons. I had a good family friend who had survived breast cancer as well, but I never had much emotional investment. It is an awesome thing to show up and see forty thousand people for one cause, but I had not been swept up in the moment. I know it was because I was there to run, and thus my competitive self took over and was more concerned about my time than why I was truly there. As I started running after surgery, I could barely make three miles. There was going to be no personal best set. My goal was just to be able to run the three point one miles.

Every year, I run for Lindsey's employer's team, rather than my own, because they have better party favors. Because life had taken over, Lindsey did not realize that the sign up date was due until a couple of days before. I sent out a note to people at my work to see if they wanted to join our team. In just those two days, I could not believe the overwhelming response from my coworkers. Again, my ignorance to the significance of my situation surfaced. They really cared! I think the difference of this race compared to the past really sunk in when the packets came and mine was full of pink shit. I had my own survivor shirt and hat. As the morning of the race dawned, I put on my pink attire and I did have a moment that it really sunk in that I was cancer free and a survivor. I was about to go out and run three point one miles, two months after having a major ass surgery. When I got downtown, though, and began to wander through the sea of pink, what I thought I would feel did not come to fruition. I guess I expected to feel some kind of kinship to others who had undergone the same journey, yet I did not. I got my pink boa, which I subsequently tied through my hat so that it would flare out behind me and went to the start line. I did not feel any emotion about the moment. Do not get me wrong. I was glad to be there, but I just was not in to it as others were. As I sit and reflect on it now, I think it was because I can count on one hand the number of times during the previous eight months when I had said, "I have cancer," and I really had not verbalized after surgery that I was cancer-free. I think it goes to my frame of mind that I refused to respect the disease. I gave it no credence, and thus felt no big release at that moment. I will say that I am very proud of the fact that I ran all three point one miles even though I wanted badly to stop, but my twelve-year-old friend was not stopping, thus my competitive ass was not going to either. I actually ran ten minute miles!

The next surgery date came up quickly. This surgery was to fix the 'dog ears' that had formed on my sides. By this point, I had no anxiety about going under the knife. I had my friend the anesthesiologist lined up to take care of me, so I had no worries. As I got my pre-surgical questions, I was in a surly mood.

As my friend asked me if I was okay, I kept joking with her how hungry I was, so every question was answered by, "Do you smell pancakes?"

The surgery lasted two hours and afterwards, I woke up in a pleasant haze. I felt somewhat nauseous, so they gave me extra medication. Apparently I also indicated I was in pain, but I do not think I was. Lindsey, who was with me, claimed I was dreaming when I said it. Thus, I got even more good stuff. The result was that I kept falling into a very deep sleep and my respiration level kept going down. So, all I remember was Lindsey continually slapping me on the shoulder and saying, "Breathe, Demmon."

I remember being very irritated with her because she was ruining my trip to my happy place. She later recounted that she plopped whatever magazine she was reading on my prone body and then occasionally would look at the monitor and slap me. I guess she did not want 'the help' to croak! I eventually did come to and spent the rest of the day pleasantly stoned at home on the couch. Of course, my ass mowed the front yard two days later and went to work after only taking the weekend off. My co-workers were bitching at me claiming that I was ruining it for everyone. How could they ever be sick if I kept coming to work so soon after having major procedures done? Much like I had been doing my whole life, I was blowing the curve for everyone else. My rationale, I thought, was reasonable because if I was to stay at home, I would just do stupid stuff there, like remodeling, more mowing, planting trees, etc. There was no harm done in my recovery, and the sides looked great. The dog ears were gone and the incision looked awesome. Two weeks later, I played my first softball game since all this began. Of course, in fine Demmon tradition, I got injured by a line drive taken off my wrist. The bruise was spectacular. I went 3 for 3 and played a stellar first base. I was back to normal.

To top off my re-entry into the world of athletics, I was asked by my friend Ann, the owner of the fabulous tiki bar, to check out dragon boat racing. A dragon boat is a forty-foot-long boat that is paddled by twenty breast cancer survivors. They race other dragon boats around the country. The best part of the whole thing is the women on the team. They are not a bunch of 'why me' type of women. They are women with attitude that did not let breast cancer define them. The first practice was a great workout and I was hooked. Normally, I hate water, but the exercise and potential for racing sang a siren song to my competitive side. I began biking to practice, paddling for an hour or so, and then biking home. About a month or so after I began practicing, I had a checkup with the oncologist. The normal routine of being felt up commenced. He began intensely probing my right armpit which was the same side as where the tumor was. I saw the frown on his face and thought, "Oh shit, here we go again."

He began asking questions about if I had noticed any changes. I had not been exactly probing my armpit on a regular basis and one does not feel resistance when applying deodorant, unless you choose the au natural route in which case I can imagine the hair causing some drag. I did tell him all about the dragon boating and that it was working my arms, but I had not noticed any other pain or discomfort. He reassured me it was probably nothing, but he nonetheless wanted me to have an ultrasound. My mind was starting to do funny things again. Despite his reassurances, I was skeptical as I knew that the data driven girl in me could not take comfort in such statements without actual proof. We all have heard 'I am sure it is probably nothing' before, so those words do not hold water for those who before found out it was something. The reassurance by the doctor was followed by 'I want it done today,' doing nothing for my confidence.

I could not get an appointment until the afternoon. I had taken the day off and was thus left to my own devices as my support system was working. I could have made various phone calls, but did not want to cause a stir over hopefully nothing. I went to my house to wait until having to go back to the doctor. The next couple of hours were spent trying not to 'go there' as I anxiously willed the clock forward. I could not work due to the mental distraction and had no motivation to start a project. In the meantime, I probed the armpit myself and did not feel anything, bolstering my confidence. At the ultrasound, the technician imaged the area for an hour. I cannot complain about their thoroughness. The doctor came in to confirm the fact that nothing was there. It turns out that all that paddling had changed the muscle structure and thus seemed to be the cause of the change felt by my oncologist. At practice that evening, I cussed out my teammates, "Damn paddling caused me a day of grief."

Later that month, I found myself standing on a shore in Atlanta waiting to participate in my first dragon boat race. It had been just over a year from my diagnosis. I stared out in the water in amazement. Could I really be getting ready to do this when just six months before I was lying in a hospital bed waking up from surgery feeling like I could just die? I stood there in the presence of over a hundred other breast cancer survivors who through their own journeys had led us all to converge in the same spot and finally felt a sense of what I had overcome. I had always shrugged off compliments from others when they said I was brave or tough. I allowed myself at that moment to say, "You know what? I am tough."

After the race, the team went back to the hotel and we partied with another dragon boat team. I stood in the corner with my drink and watched the group. I continued to marvel at the resolve of the human being. We were celebrating life, not being victims. After talking to several of the women, my decision to document my story was reinforced as I continued to listen to others who had the same feeling during their cancer journey of not having the pertinent information to make informed decisions during their treatment. If I help ease the path for just one person, then I consider this a work of art!

The Icing on the Cake

THE TIME TO GET NIPPLES had arrived. There are choices with respect to your headlights. You can get the areole and nipples tattooed and be done with it, or you can have a three dimensional reconstruction done. There are a couple of options with the 3D approach. One is that they fold the existing skin into a nipple—kind of like Origami—or they transplant skin from another area, usually your inner thigh, to make the nipple. If considering 3D construction, remember that skin that is transplanted from other parts of the body comes with hair follicles. In other words, you need to ask if you will end up having pubes on your boobs—hey, it rhymes. There are methods to remove the hair, but I was not too thrilled with the prospect of having yet another hair area to maintain. So I elected to go with the Origami option. I had a challenge, however, to find yet another plastic surgeon. I had made the decision not to go back to New York to get this part completed. The main reason was expenses. If I were to return to New York, I would have to pay for the flight and then another week's stay. As much as I loved the senior assisted living facility, I did not want to take the time away from my work. So I began the process of finding a plastic surgeon that would be willing to complete someone else's work.

I did not have to look very hard. I had heard of a surgeon in Indianapolis that had just trained on the DIEP. He knew of my plight through my anesthesiologist. He had no problem finishing the reconstruction. At my consultation, he was great and explained the procedure very well using visual props—scissors and a piece of paper. Since I was numb, the surgery was to be performed while I was awake with just a local anesthetic. You can have something to relax you, if you choose. Since I was a fan of being relaxed, I chose this option. I did not want to relive the whole biopsy episode over again—"sure you'll be numb—you won't feel a thing . . . " The surgeon came into pre-op, performed measurements and showed me where he was going to put the nipples.

Lindsey, as usual, was my ride, and was 'helping' by asking him, "You are going to be measuring twice, aren't you?" 'You know, measure twice, cut once.'

I agreed with where he indicated to place the nipples, and was then whisked off to the operating room for what I hoped would be my last surgery. I hopped up on the table and the nurses scrubbed me off with betadine to sterilize the area. The operating room was freezing, but my hot flashes came in handy. One of the nurses had great tunes playing, so once they infused some Versed, I was a happy camper. They placed a drape over my face and I drifted in a nice place between almost asleep and consciousness. Now the thing about Versed is that it lowers your inhibitions. A Prince song came on and I heard one of the nurses tell how they once went on stage with him.

They asked what song he sang and she said, "It was 'Little Red Corvette.' "

Me, being the naughty individual, was thinking of one of his racier tunes.

The plastic surgeon, whilst sewing on my nipples said, "That wasn't the song I was thinking of."

"Me neither," I replied.

"Well what song were you thinking of?" he asked.

"Well", I replied, "It has cussing so I can't sing it."

The surgeon said, "I bet we are thinking of the same song. Come on and sing it and I will sing along."

Me, being under the influence of Versed, started belting out in a high, Prince-like wail, "You Sexy Mother Fucker."

To give him credit, he sang along with me, word for word. The procedure took just about an hour. I went home with two large bandages on the girls and no idea what they looked like.

My instructions were not to shower for three days and to not wear a bra for two weeks. Being the sadist, I went to work the next day looking like I had two packs of cigarettes attached to the front of my boobs. No conversation at work over the next two days occurred with direct eye contact. The staring was shameless. It was like Christmas when I took the bandages off to finally see my new headlights. They looked very realistic. I was very pleased.

Tattooing is the last step for 3D nipples to make the coloring darker. I had several suggestions from those that I am sure care deeply about me to have skulls tattooed or some other objects instead of just filling in the color. Had I not been single, I would have considered doing something funky. The plastic surgeon's office had a tattoo artist that would be performing the act.

Full Circle

THE TIME HAD COME FOR my annual visit back to my family doctor. I sat and thought the night before what I would say. I had not talked to him since I had been diagnosed. I knew that he had been getting records and I had listed all the procedures that I done over the year. He walked into the room and said, "Wow, you have been through a lot over the past year. Let's talk about it."

"First, how are you doing?" he asked.

"I am doing well," I replied.

He then said, "How's your support system?"

I was laughing on the inside, thinking, "Well, they are all jack assess!" But I replied instead, "I have a great support system." I then recapped in about five minutes the events of the past year.

He asked, "What do you think could have been done differently?"

I was taken aback and pleasantly surprised. He was soliciting the exact information that I wanted to impart to him.

I said, "Well, first, I wish that we had been more aggressive when the calcium deposits were observed in the first mammogram and sought alternate imaging."

Notice that I did say we. As I have said throughout this entire sordid tale, I do believe that the patient needs to be more aggressive when it comes to their own health care. I then told him that I had learned throughout this process that I believe that mammograms are not sufficient when a patient presents with fibrocystic breasts. He was receptive to the message.

I wasn't expecting an, "Oh yes, you are absolutely right. Ultrasounds and MRI's for everyone!" We both agreed that my initial presentation led us both to complacency.

He then said, "You know that both you and I will spend a lot of time racking our brains on what we both could have done differently."

Those are the words I really wanted to hear. He was acknowledging that he wanted to learn from the experience as well.

We spoke for almost an hour. It was a great, honest talk. During the course of the conversation, I also indicated what had happened to the first surgeon that I saw. This subject led to a conversation about the patient and doctor interaction. I stated that I believed that in this day and age with the internet, the patient is more informed. Some become dangerous with their access to knowledge, but their questions are valid all the same. A doctor needs to take a different approach with patients. In the past, patients came in and accepted what the doctor told them. Now, patients come armed with information and are more engaged in their care. I did say that I realize that this can be a pain in the ass for doctors as a patient comes in already self-diagnosed and may tell the doctor what they need. There needs to be a happy medium where the patient is allowed to question the doctor without the physician becoming defensive and where the doctor can still be recognized as the health care authority. I wanted him to know that a doctor must not become defensive when questioned. This makes the patient feel like they have done something wrong. In the end, as my friend Lisa says, a patient just wants to be taken seriously and wants to be heard. He did agree that doctors need to adapt to today's patient.

I left feeling wistful. It was ironic that two weeks shy of the one year anniversary of being diagnosed, I had finally achieved some closure.

Leggo My Eggo

AT MY THIRD CHECK-UP with my oncologist since surgery, I was asked by the doctor about my hot flashes and how I was dealing with them. I had already turned him down at previous visits on taking anti-depressants, a common treatment for hot flashes in women who cannot take hormone therapy. I just did not believe in taking them when I was not depressed. I know of their side effects and would rather suffer through the sweating. I did mention that I could feel my hormones cycle each month as I neared the time for my shot. My ovaries were trying to rebel. My oncologist asked me if I had given a second thought to having my ovaries removed. In truth, I had. The previous month I was five days late for my shot and experienced slight premenstrual syndrome and break-through bleeding. I also felt a little sick that week as well. This did alarm me because it indicated the strength of my hormones. The thought of another surgery, though, did not set well with me. I was tired of the process of having my body recover from trauma. I felt like over the past year, when I would work myself up physically and feel pretty good, I would have some procedure done that would knock me back down again. The only incentive was that I was maxed out on my insurance.

My oncologist indicated that after discussion with his peers, the general consensus was that there was a better outcome long term if the ovaries were removed. This information combined with the previous month's hormone swings were enough to finally convince me to do the deed. I now had to find yet another surgeon to rip out my ovaries. Using my connections,

I quickly found an gynecologist to remove more organs—no I had not been neglecting my naughty bits—I had my general doctor check those parts out on a regular basis. The surgeon I found was great. Previously, my general doctor had asked me to consider the full hysterectomy. I figured, "Hell, why not get everything yanked out if I am not going to use it." However, at my visit to the obstetrician, he challenged having the cervix and uterus removed. The doctor indicated that cervical and uterine cancers are much easier to detect than ovarian. What I did not think about is that at the end of my Arimidex therapy, I could still accept a donor egg, if I so chose in the future. I informed the general public that I would be interviewing possible donors. I know it will be hard to find someone with better genes than myself, but, if five years down the road I decide to conceive a child naturally, I will have to make that concession. In the end, I went ahead and left the cervix and the uterus. I really do not think I want to get pregnant at the age of forty-three, but at least I will have the option.

In an unusual twist, I found myself scheduled for surgery on the same day in the same hospital as my aunt, who was having a full hysterectomy. I had it arranged so that the same anesthesiologist was performing the surgery. As usual, Lindsey drove me to get sliced. The surgery was outpatient, so I got to go home the same day. The surgery took about an hour. I was disappointed, however, because the surgeon tried to go in through my belly button to perform the surgery laproscopically, but because it had been reconstructed, he could not maneuver well, so had to make additional incisions in my side. That was the only hiccup with the procedure, so I inherited yet more visible battle scars. I only took a week off of work. The pain was more than I expected, and in retrospect, I should have asked for more time, but I am a sadist. I can say that the pain was worth it as I will no longer have to worry about ovarian cancer and my hormones can now surrender their war in my body.

My Tramp Stamps

A WEEK AFTER THE REMOVAL of my ovaries, the time came to get my areoles tattooed. I was very excited as this marked the last step of the reconstruction process. The tattoo is applied by a nurse practitioner that is typically associated with a plastic surgeon and takes a little over an hour. The nurse called me up prior to the appointment to ask about coloring. I stalled at this question as I had trouble remembering what color they were. Were they a brown or pink shade? I honestly could not remember. Who pays attention to these things? I settled on a shade—I will not tattoo and tell...—and showed up for my appointment. Not ever having a tattoo before, I had no idea on how the process worked. I knew from others that had gotten tattoos that they hurt, but I was not concerned about pain as the area was numb. That comfort was soon dispelled as the nurse injected numbing medication in the area and it hurt. I thought, "What the hell, I am supposed to be numb there!"

The nurse indicated that this is a common thought among women that are getting the tattoo and that in fact they will feel pain. I was definitely caught off guard. Let me be the first to tell you, it hurts like hell. I cannot understand why someone would voluntarily get one of these, especially since when you normally get a tattoo, you are not numbed at all, and I have seen some pictures of tattoos in some sensitive places. I have been told that tattoos are addictive; however, I don't get it. Regardless, she completed the tattoo, even putting on the Montgomery glands—those little bumps you have on your areola and nipple. For the next week, I had to treat the area with Vaseline and keep it covered. It takes two months for the color to appear what it will be permanently. A touch up may be required if the ink doesn't take. Needless to say, I am very happy with the outcome. A person really couldn't tell the difference if it weren't for the mammogram scars. Hopefully, they will fade with time.

Lessons Learned

THE MOST COMMON THINGS THAT I HEAR or read from people with cancer is to ask "Why me?" and to thank the disease. I cannot bring myself to do either of those things. Why not me? If my getting this disease meant that someone else close to me does not have it, then great. Would I change my mind about this statement if my experience was worse or if my condition was terminal? No. I believe that the good Lord has a destiny for all of us and it is up to us to live it. Could I have done something different in my earlier years to prevent this from happening to me? Maybe. But is that not true of normal life? Do we not always look back and wish we had done this or that? So, I do not regret the choices that I made in the past because they helped define who I am.

As far as thanking the disease, I find this very odd. I think that people who thank the disease were not happy with themselves before the cancer. They thank cancer for coming out the side a different person. I am not saying that this process has not changed me. There are lessons to be learned here. But my very core, I believe has not changed. I was happy with pre-cancer Sarah, for the most part. I was successful in my career (and still am), I was giving to others (and hope I still am), I had great family and friends (and still do) and was doing what I wanted. I am not mad at cancer for disrupting the flow of my life, more like very irritated. But I am a firm believer in looking at every life situation for improvement for myself, and cancer is no exception.

So what have I discovered or learned from this experience? I learned that I must be actively engaged in my own health. I cannot become complacent when I think there is something wrong. I must listen to my body and most importantly pay attention to my instincts. I think I knew deep down that this lump was different than the others. I think my friends knew as well. But when pressed about it, I would always say, "Oh I am sure it is a fibroid."

My friends fed off of my reassurance that everything was okay. I also fed off of telling myself it was nothing. I did not press the doctor when deep in some core, I knew I should have. I am not saying I will become a hypochondriac after this experience, but I will pay more attention to things that I feel are not right.

I have learned to have more patience, except in the car where my language has remained as colorful as ever—I mean, I have had a double mastectomy for the love of God, yet I can lift my arm up to use the turn signal…. When I observe someone who looks different, I find myself engaging the person. For example, I rode in the hospital elevator with a teen confined to a wheelchair with an obvious severe birth defect. Instead of trying to look everywhere but at him and ride in silence, as we are all taught to do by our parents—it is not polite to stare, you know,—I smiled and said hello and asked him how it was going. This was a major feat for my normally introverted self anyway, but having been stared at unmercifully for months, I know what I wanted those people to do. Just nod and smile. It is not wrong to look, just do not pity me. Treat me normal. That is all I asked of those who knew me when I started this journey.

Cancer gave me an extra boost of self confidence, along with the tummy tuck and the new hooters! While I maintain an outer core that everyone perceives as not caring what others think, I am just as insecure as the next person. The outpouring of support from people that I did not even really know that well opened my eyes to the kind of impact I was having in this world. I also learned that it is okay to accept help from others. I do not have to continually demonstrate my independence to the world.

They know I am successful and can wire my own lighting. It is okay to be vulnerable. The world will not look upon it as weak. I will always have to temper this urge, but I have become more cognizant of it. As I write this, I am waiting for Oprah or Dr. Phil to bust in the door.

Did I need cancer to realize any of these things? No, just a night of liquor and deep thinking. But to test your interactions and relationships with others in the confines of normal life is a hard, scary thing to do, because of the fear of rejection. There is a fear that all that you bring to the table will not be reciprocated. You have to get over that fear. Understand that if you believe and trust, you will be taken care of. You can never prepare for this disease, but you can invest in your life such that if you are diagnosed with cancer, you have the tools and support to fight it.

The Emails

08/28/2007:

So in the spirit of blogging, I am sending this message to a large group of people because it has become cumbersome to keep up on work and updates (no offense to anyone, I am very overwhelmed at the support that all of you have offered and believe me I will come knocking on some of your doors.) I also keep forgetting who I have told and who I have not. Finally, many of you need to know from the standpoint that I may be telecommuting throughout the upcoming ordeal and that obviously will affect my working relationship with you.

To recap, I was diagnosed with breast cancer two weeks ago. I have undergone a series of screens, through a couple of doctors and am ready to attack this thing. I will be going to IU to a great surgeon and one of their top oncologists. I will be doing an aggressive course of treatment due to my age and fitness level, so I will begin chemo next week. In two weeks, I will be Telly Savalas reincarnate. To prepare you all, I think you know that I am not a wig sort of girl, so I am going the do-rag route, so if you find any that are obnoxious and fit my personality, send them my way. Thanks to Pam for her trip to the Harley shop already! I have a good prognosis so far. Chest X-rays are negative, by feel there appears to be no lymph involvement, but the tumor is quite large, so after chemo, surgery will be needed and there is a good chance of having to lose it. So for the next three months, I will be in and out of the office sporadically. If you need to schedule a meeting with me, you may want to make telecon arrangements along with it in case I am working from home that day. My goal is to maintain as normal a lifestyle as I can, but I do realize that I will need to rest as well and as the course of chemo progresses, so does the fatigue. I have also found out that the drugs cause you to possibly become scatter brained, (I know, insert joke here) so if I have not responded to a request in my usual timely manner, I will take no offense in reminders.

Cindy and Sacha are always in the loop, so if you really need to know something, and I am not around, then you can ask them. Also, for project needs, if you need something urgent, Cathy will be my back up.

Finally, I would hope that you all would continue to harass me as you normally would. You all know my sense of humor and will act accordingly.

I will try to send updates when I know more. I only have one more piece of the puzzle that I will receive today. If you do not want to be on this list, please let me know. I will not take offense.

09/10/2007:

Someone put out a new blog, so I cannot be outdone! Well, my first chemo was last Tuesday. Normally they would be on Mondays, but because of the holiday, I got moved to Tuesday. As you all are probably not aware, Tuesday is primarily testes day at the chemo clinic. That is when the patients of Lance Armstrong's doctor come in for their treatment. Much to my disappointment, however, there were not any hot dudes, but only old men. Much to my delight, when I walked back to the chemo lounge for the first time to have a test done—you will all be relieved to know that I am not pregnant for anyone sweating that detail—and there was a volunteer there playing the harp for the patients receiving chemo. As most of you know, my music choice tends to be a little harder than the harp, so I quickly informed my nurse that I would prefer being seated in a different section where it didn't sound like a funeral home. Don't get me wrong, I appreciate those that want to volunteer, but in the spirit of heal-ing, I would like my music a little more upbeat. I don't know if she knew any Billy Idol, so maybe I just didn't give her enough *time. Thankfully she was gone by the time I got strapped in the chair.*

The actual infusion takes about one and a half hours. First they infuse anti-nausea stuff, and then it is fifteen minutes of the first chemo drug (which is bright red and yes, you get to experience that later) then forty-five minutes of the other. Then they send you on your way. I am looking at only five more to go, instead of eleven weeks to go.

The side effects have mainly been an underlying vertigo, headache and fatigue. No nausea as of yet. The day after chemo, I have to give myself an injection of a drug called Neulasta that regenerates your white blood cells that the chemo kills. Anyway, the side effect is you feel like the flu twenty-four hours after. I felt fine on Thursday thinking I was in the clear until Friday about 3pm. I believe every lymph node in my body became swollen. Needless to say, Friday night and Sat. through the afternoon were spent on the couch. Thankfully, the symptoms only lasted those twenty-four hours.

If you haven't seen the new do, I think I may be keeping it, unless people are just being nice, which doesn't happen much with you, people. I got it cut real short to ease the transition to the inevitable of the hair falling out. I now have an IU do-rag thanks to Cole, a lovely set of Harley do-rags and a wicked skull do-rag from Kevin R.

That is the update for now. Thanks again for all your thoughts and prayers. The true test will be how the body handles the cumulative effect as the next treatment is next Monday.

09/18/2007:

Treatment number two was Monday. I did find out that I have two other treatments I didn't factor in, so six more to go. I got yelled at for digging a hole and planting a tree which caused my arm to swell. I defended myself by telling them that I was allowed to do normal activity, but their idea of normal and mine is obviously different. Oh, well.

The hair started falling out yesterday, so it was officially shaved last evening. It was somewhat traumatic right after I did it, but was reassured I had a cute head. It is do-rag city for now on.

Otherwise, the treatment went well. No harps this time. I did ask her if they could have Matthew McConaughey come and play the harp, but it was no dice on my request. What kind of place are they running anyway?

That is all the update for now. Another week of feeling like booty. The good thing is that the week after I feel pretty good, so that helps. Only two more treatments of the harsh stuff.

10/04/2007:

Well, the past two weeks have been fun. So we pick up our cancer adventure after the arm swelling, tree planting, and stump removal incident. Later that week, after injecting myself with the Neulasta shot, my arm swelled again. I went ahead, because you know that is how I roll with my work, because I am a martyr. Well, on Friday, after two days of swelling and some yelling from certain individuals, I let the surgeon know what was going on— mind you, I already told her about this earlier in the week, had a Doppler to look at my veins which were negative, so this is not the first time she heard about this in my defense—and she sent me back Friday afternoon for another Doppler. Next thing I know I am getting admitted to the hospital because the first crack-smoking technician, earlier in the week, failed to detect the blood clot in my clavicle reducing the blood flow to my jugular. Was that why I felt dizzy? They took me into surgery that evening and removed my port and I now am on two blood thinners—I apparently excel at everything, including clotting. Well, that gets injected twice a day in my gut, so the bruises I have are very spectacular. I had a PICC line put in last Thursday for my treatment on Monday, which meant a lovely tube flopping around my bicep just ready to catch on things.

Treatment was Monday, where they took the PICC line out. This time there were no harps, banjos, but an offer to take a mosaic class where we can talk about our feelings and then solidify them by gluing pieces of glass together. I felt pretty rough yesterday and slept for most of it, as I rode the Neulasta wave. I feel better today. I will get a new port next Friday, this time in my jugular. Since it is bigger it will have reduced risk of getting a clot around it, or else I just have a stroke that much quicker.

The oncologist indicated that the tumor seems to have reduced by 0.5 cm and feels mushier, which is good. I am, by the way, charging $10 for anyone that wants to touch the tumor. That way I can meet my HRA bridge.

Some disappointing news from today—hot off the presses— is that the plastic surgeon doesn't want to do immediate recon- struction. There apparently is a high risk of deformity due to the radiation treatment's effect on the skin, so I may have to wait six months to a year post mastectomy to get new girls. This will give all you volunteers—you know who you are, lest I tell your wives—a chance to really evaluate your choices for the new ones. I am not happy about this new piece of information, but will of course have to do what they say in the best interest of getting the ultimate outcome that I want.

10/23/2007:

I have had an adventurous last week or two, so my apologies to my legions of fans who enjoy the tumor blog and were expect- ing this sooner. So I went into surgery on Oct. 12th to have a new port installed. When I woke up two hours later, I had three new incisions and no new port. Apparently the way that my veins branch, it makes port placement blind very difficult. Complicat- ing the fact that I started bleeding—due to the Clydesdale size dose of blood thinner that I am on, no doubt,—they decided to stop. Glue a bolt on either side of my neck and my Halloween outfit is complete as I look like I got in a knife fight at the local Harley bar. So, I went into interventional radiology on the fol- lowing Monday to give it another try. They did a crappy job of placing the port, so it sits as a big lump on my chest. To make it more enjoyable, I had to have chemo the next day on the bruised spot. Needless to say I rode the vicodin train for the rest of the week. To make matters worse, the incision was such that every- time I dared to move my right arm, the sutures would bust open and bleed. I spent every day but one last week at some hospital. Anyone going through my trash at home would have thought a homicide took place in my house due to the copious amount of bloody bandages. After putting a compression bandage on and sending me home to pass out on Thursday, they were finally able to get the bleeding under control. I can only pray for the bruising to be less next Monday for chemo, otherwise, more pain.

The tumor—I think we should have a contest to name it—has shrunk an additional 0.5 cm. I reached the halfway point last week in my treatment. I will now start a course of eight weeks of Taxol. The possible side effects are different and include neuropathy (tingling or numbness in the extremities), feeling like you are arthritic, hair loss (already there), possible allergic reaction to the chromaphore in the formulation, and having your fingernails and toenails turn ugly yellow and pop off. Nausea is not supposed to be an issue with this drug. The infusion time is long (three hours) so that gives me more quality time with the harpist (who incidentally was at the last session and drove my aunt batty.)

As most of you can guess, I will not be having my annual Halloween party this year. Just too much for me to do right now. I am considering a Saturday party in the not so distant future when the leaves are dropped where if you come with your rake and do my leaves, I may serve food and alcohol. Stay tuned for that. That is all the excitement for now.

11/30/2007:

I haven't sent one of these in a while and have gotten reminded of the fact, so here is my latest and greatest in the world of tumors and ports. Seven treatments down and one to go. I had my latest one on Monday. I am now on Taxol and happy to report that I still have all my fingernails and toe nails and no neuropathy. However, I do have the joy of the arthralgia which can best be described as having growing pains in my legs. And the best part is that I now have hot flashes at night—for all the wrong reasons. The pain in my legs lasts from Tuesday to about Sunday, so I still have a good week in between treat-

ments. My last treatment is Dec. 10th. I will actually go in that afternoon immediately following chemo to have surgery to take this damn port out. It has been the bane of my existence for this whole time. So, other than being a hot menopausal thirty-seven year old, things are going well.

As for the big surgery, things have changed there as well. I went to consult with a plastic surgeon on my options for recon-struction. She was very negative and basically did not want to do anything to me because I wanted to maintain my quality of living with respect to being able to continue to do sports half way competitively—I have delusions of grandeur that I am actually half way decent at softball, golf, etc. The literature and the surgeon suggest that implants are not a viable option for someone that undergoes radiation post mastectomy because the skin gets damaged. That leaves only two options, at least in our great state of Indiana, of the TRAM flap where they cut your abdominal muscles, or the lattissimus flap where they cut your back muscle, leaving you with only your rib muscles. Everything I have read so far and from those I have spoken to points to serious permanent loss of strength. In some cases, people can-not even lift their arms over their heads. This left me in quite the dilemma. She mentioned another procedure that I had read about called DIEP, but didn't say much about it and didn't give me a starting point. I did some surfing and found a doctor in New York that has done eight hundred of these. The procedure is less invasive and does not destroy muscle. I emailed the guy and he actually called me at home at 9:30 at night. I was impressed. I am flying out there next week to consult with him. My general surgeon here is very supportive and thinks it is also the best option for me. The best part is that I can have reconstruction done immediately instead of having to wait. If I have surgery there, I will only be gone for two weeks. He has had marathon-ers, kayakers and other athletes undergo this successfully. All in all, things are looking up. My surgeon this week even suggested that depending on the pathology post surgery, I may not need radiation. I am not getting my hopes up, but it would be nice.

Thanks for everyone's inquiries into my leaf situation. My sister and brother-in-law were down for a wedding so they did the majority of them for me. I only have two trees that are hanging on. I think I can manage that debris! Stay tuned for a post work outing the week of Dec. 17th. Of course I will be a cheap date, but a happy one!

1/28/2007:

I have been negligent in my updating to my devote followers of a tale of two—okay, rhymes with cities. I have gotten a lot of questions about surgery, so here is the scoop.

For those of you who have not seen me since Christmas, I have ditched the do-rag and am sporting a good start on the hair growth. Now I look like a GI Jane devotee. I am now going to start charging for petting my head. I feel great and have been working out. I can run three miles now. The first day I tried to run, I could only go about a mile and was thoroughly pissed off until I had to remind myself that I did just go through four months of chemo.

My surgery is next Tuesday in New York City. Actually Long Island. I leave Monday morning. The nervousness currently is flying with my mother who is sporting two frankenboots (you know, those lovely things they put on your legs when they have fractures) and has not flown since 1996. We will have to dump her bag out and look for sharp objects and lotions and creams. I may have to be heavily medicated before I even arrive. I have a whole entourage coming, so I will have a lot of people to take care of my nappy arse. I will be getting the double mastectomy followed by immediate reconstruction with the new procedure that I had described before. The surgery can be up to eighteen hours because there are a lot of blood vessels to move around. But no muscle to cut (only as a last resort,) so it will be worth it to me. And I get all the fat taken out of my gut. I did ask about taking the fat out of my posterior, of which I have plenty, but those of you who are blessed like me to have copious amounts of fat there know that it is rather lumpy and it would be lumpy in the front too. Alas, I only get rid of the belly (and no, I am not accepting donations.)

I will have to remain in Long Island until the 14th. I supposedly get out of the hospital the 8th and will then relocate to a nearby hotel.

My current plan is to take the rest of February off and come back in March. For those of you needing project help, Cathy will be large and in charge. I hope I have gotten everybody set before I leave, so I apologize if I forgot something. I am sure that it will be fine, but you all know how neurotic I am about being in control!

Cindy and Sacha will get info after the surgery, so I will have them send out a message that I made it through with flying colors. Hopefully when I get back to the hotel, I will be off the narcotics enough to send email—Friends, don't let friends send emails under the influence.

I also found out last week that three to four weeks post surgery I will indeed be getting radiation. That is six weeks, every day except for weekends. I anticipate working through that period. I will have a minor reconstruction performed in three to four months, then hopefully this will be a distant memory.

2/11/2008:

Yes it is an email from Frankenstein to inform you that I am back among the living. I finally was able to get a wifi connection—and to walk to a room that has it, more importantly—and had a window of opportunity where I didn't need a nappy.

As you can see from Cindy's emails, everything went well with the surgery. I am a mass of drainage tubes and stitches, but more importantly, I am now cancer free. The gory blow by blow is as follows:

I went into surgery on Tuesday at 7:30am and came out about 11pm. I briefly remember waking up in a haze, vomiting and passing back out. I spent most of Wednesday in ICU, in a morphine-induced haze because, let me tell you, I was in the worst pain in my life. I was okay if I died that day because I was sincerely miserable. For any of you considering a tummy tuck, think twice. They moved me to a room on Wednesday afternoon where I tried to eat pineapple. They then tried to sit me up in a chair which resulted in more vomiting, crying and proficient use of the 'f' word. At that point I could not move without assistance, but got up a couple of times with their help. Meanwhile, I was being poked or prodded about once an hour. On Thursday, they decided to remove the catheter, resulting in me having to page the nurse every so often to help me up. To get up took several minutes and good use of my verbal skills as a sailor. I hope I didn't scar them for life. My doctor came in late on Thursday night and asked if I had gotten up on my own yet. I had not, but took that as a cue to get my ass up and moving. So about 2am, I did make it up by myself. It was a small but significant victory, as that was yet another step towards independence. On Thursday, they also took away my PCA pump (with the morphine) which I was very sad about. They replaced it with percocet, which does pretty good too, but I only got that for the day. Friday morning they kicked me out of the hospital and back to my digs.

For those of you who didn't know, I had a hotel all set up for my visit. Before I left I called the doctor to tell them about my arrangements. They called back to inform me that the hotel was one that charged by the hour. I thus was in a panic for the next two days trying to find a hotel where I didn't have to work off my rent (although I was conveniently lying down already . . .) The doctor came up with an agreement with a senior assisted living facility. Before you all laugh, the place has been great to both me and my family. They have these little apartments, a driver that takes you to the doctor and a whole host of characters that I have yet to meet, but my family has become well acquainted with. I think my family has gotten a kick (although none will admit it in case we consider sending them there permanently) out of the joint and the town. My uncle especially enjoyed the area and all the people. He and my mom left me yesterday in the capable hands of my aunt and cousin, although I am doing pretty good on my own. I cannot dress myself yet, and I have eight drains hanging out of me making movement not so fun. It is a fashion statement where I decide to store them for the day. I will leave out the rest of those details about emptying them and measuring except that at least I get to do some science while I am here.

Some short family funnies are as follows: Mom lost control of her wheel chair in her stubbornness to not wait and rolled into, thankfully, stopped traffic; I had to wheel her, two checked bags her checked bag and my carry on through the airport resulting in a torn finger and the start of my back problems. My adventurous uncle decided to take the bus back one night from the hospital with mom in the wheel chair. They only missed one stop, but there was some unhappiness I detected there. Alcohol was involved Friday night and there was some concern by mom over getting appropriately wheeled back by the family. They asked the tavern owner if they were incapable if he would, and he said of course. She then came back and complained about the alcoholics in the family, which is very funny to me since I would have been right there with them if I could. My cousin and aunt were stopped yesterday to be on a TV show—Gordon Ramsey from Hell's kitchen—but it involved them getting in a car with some stranger at the drug store. I think it was someone trying to abduct them.

Today is the first day where I have been awake most of the day. It gets hard being in the same position and unable to roll over, so my back is on fire as well. I am trying not to use the pain killers because I am of the philosophy that I will get better faster without them. Others may disagree. In the night I have to use them to sleep, but during the day, the discomfort is not so bad that I need to keep popping them.

As for the results of the surgery, everything looks great. The doctor seems pleased with the outcome. It is hard to tell because of all the stitches and drains, but what I can tell, it does look good. The best news was about the nature of the tumor as it appears to have been totally confined and not in any muscle or lymph nodes. Final pathology results are next week. I hope to get these drains out on Thursday, before I leave. I am under a lot of disbelief how quickly the human body rebounds. I don't know how older people, especially if they are not in shape, recover *from open heart surgery, for example, because I thought I was tough until I woke up on Wednesday.*

I will try to send out more updates this week. I wanted to thank everyone again for their get-well wishes and to Clay and Carissa for the flowers. I will be back before you know it.

Hopefully I will have wifi in my room by tomorrow, although the walking trip is good and probably needed.

Glossary —
By No Means Wikipedia

THIS IS A LIST OF TERMS that you will hear, defined in my own simple terms.

Ductile: Located in the milk ducts of the breast.

Invasive Ductile: The cancer started in the milk duct, but now has spread outside of the duct. DO NOT PANIC. This is the most common form of breast cancer and invasive does not always equal spreading outside the breast.

TRAM: Trans Rectus Abdominus Muscle. The muscle that runs down the center of your belly. Reconstruction option that involves cutting this muscle and using it to reconstruct the breast.

DIEP: Deep Inferior Epigastric Perforator. It refers to the reconstruction option where the belly fat and overlying blood vessels are used to reconstruct the breast. No muscle is cut.

Latissimus: Your upper back muscle. A reconstruction option is to cut this muscle and bring it around to the front to reconstruct the breast.

ACT: Adriamycin plus Cytoxan, followed by Taxol. Common course of chemotherapy.

Adriamycin: Also called Doxorubicin. A chemotherapy drug that treats a wide variety of cancers.

Cytoxan: A chemotherapy drug.

Taxol: A chemotherapy drug.

Tamoxifen: Drug that modulates estrogen. Used as a long-term treatment for estrogen positive breast cancers.

Aromatase Inhibitor: Drug that reduces the production of estrogen. Used as a long-term treatment for estrogen positive breast cancers.

MAC-Sedation: Monitored Anesthesia Care. A method of sedation where the patient does not require intubation.

Dose Dense: An aggressive treatment form of chemo where typically the individual is dosed every other week.

Lumpectomy: Removal of the lump only. Sometimes called breast conserving surgery.

Mastectomy: Removal of the breast. There are two types: A simple mastectomy is the removal of the breast tissue. A radical mastectomy removes both the breast tissue and some or all of the lymph nodes under the arm.

Bilateral: Both sides, as in a bilateral mastectomy.

In situ: The tumor is contained within a lobe or duct and has not spread to the surrounding tissue.

Lobular: Lobular cancer is when the cancer is located in the lobes of the breast rather than the ducts. Your breast is made up of several lobes. The milk ducts run to the lobes.

HER2: Gene that is over expressed in some breast cancers.

ER: Estrogen Receptor. Some tumors are estrogen receptor positive meaning they feed off of the estrogen in your body.

References

"Be a Survivor" by Vladimir Lange

http://www.breastcancer.org/

http://www.breastflap.com/

http://www.nationalbreastcancer.org/

http://cms.komen.org/komen/index.htm/

http://www.tube-ez.com/

"Breast Cancer Survival Manual, Fourth Edition: A Step-by-Step Guide for the Woman with Newly Diagnosed Breast Cancer", by John Link

The Photo Montage

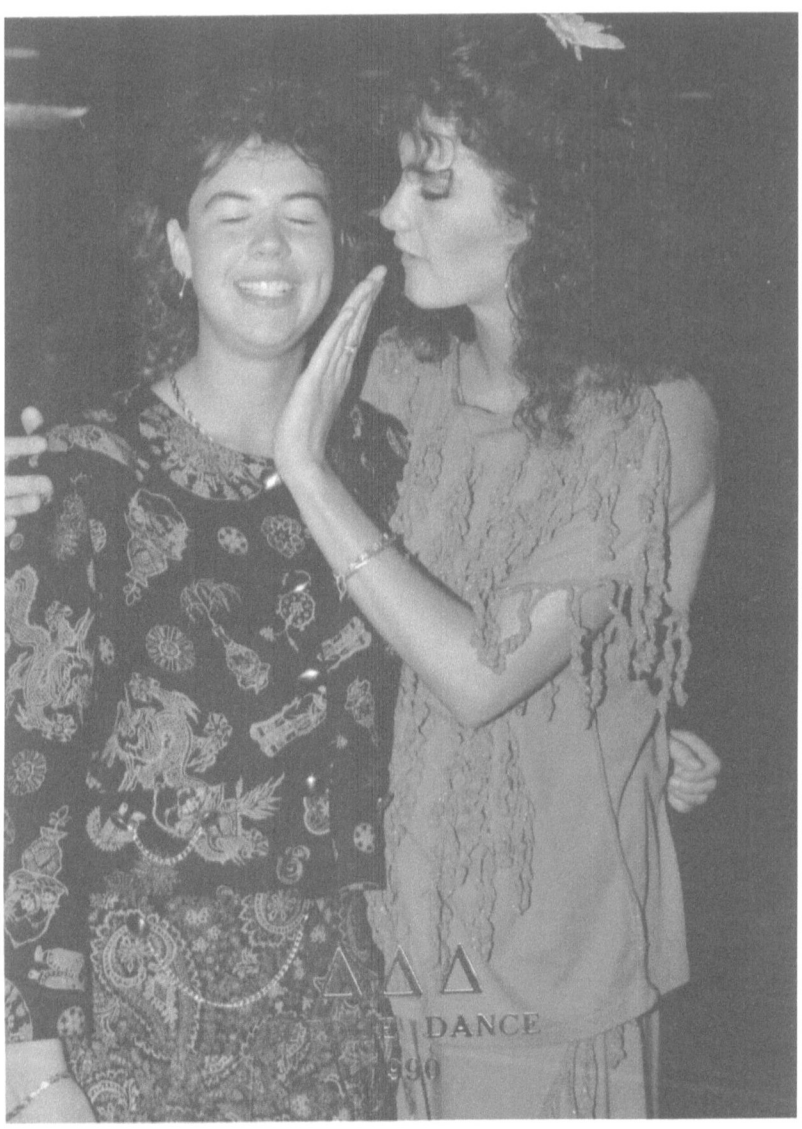

Lindsey (on the right) and I at a sorority dance (1990). She was a Jackass from Day 1. Check out my MC Hammer outfit and mall hair. I was stylin'!

106

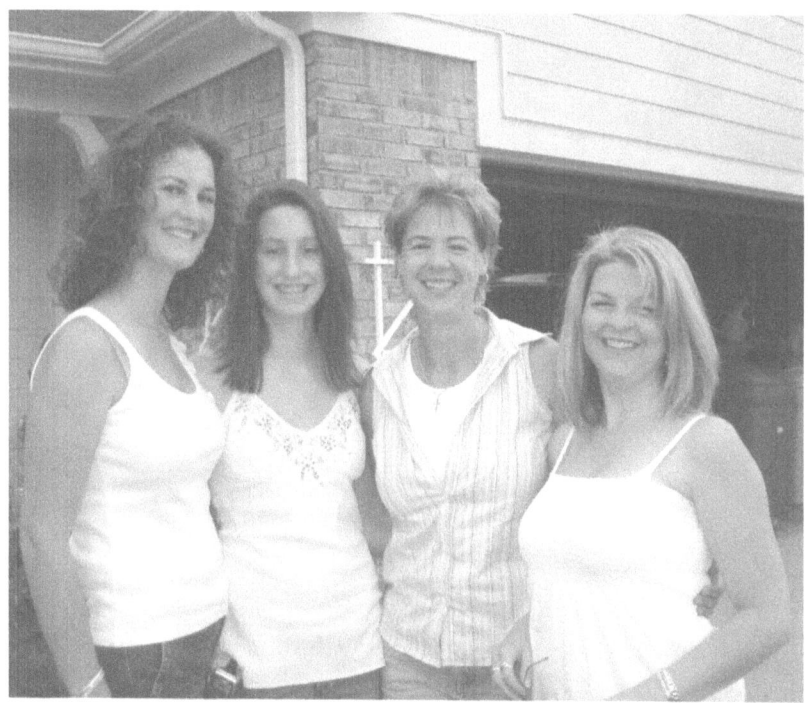

From left to right: Lindsey, her daughter Sydney, me and Ginger prior to attending a Coldplay concert. This was exactly a year before my diagnosis. I had trained hard for the Indianapolis mini marathon that year and was looking fine.

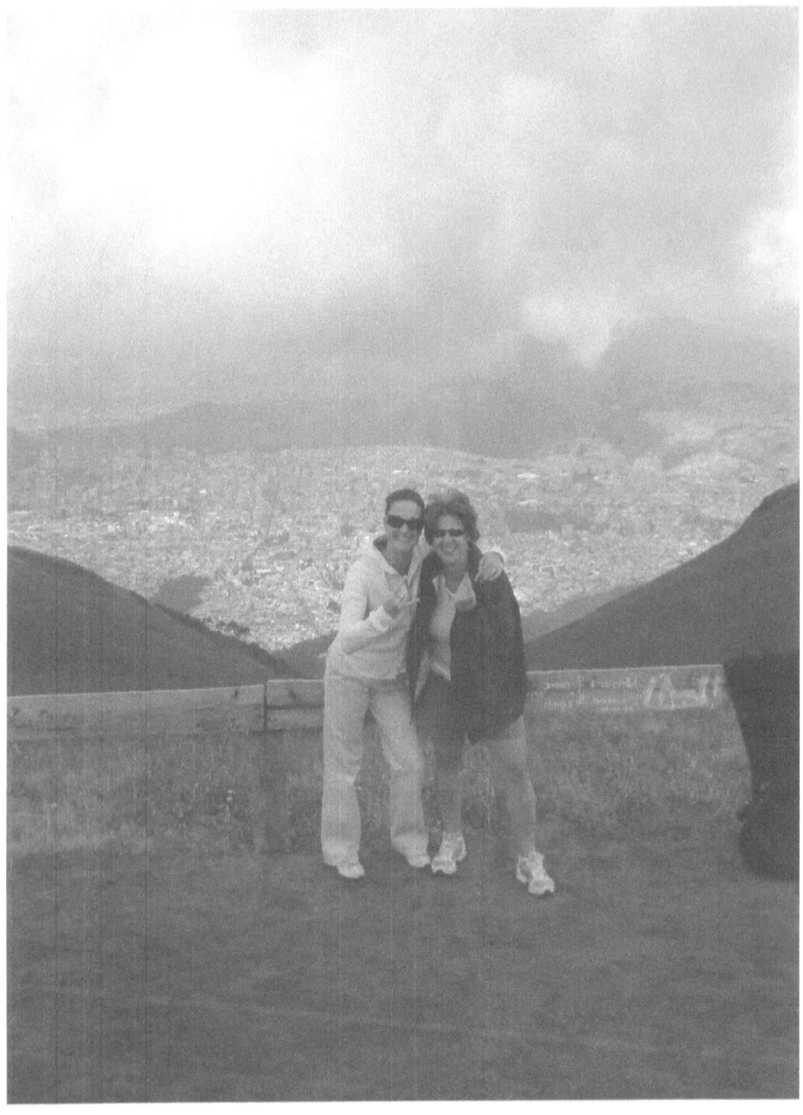

Lindsey and I on a mountain in Ecuador. We were attending her brother's wedding. This was taken just a little over three weeks before my diagnosis. How ironic I was making Rock and Roll fingers as my world was about to be rocked.

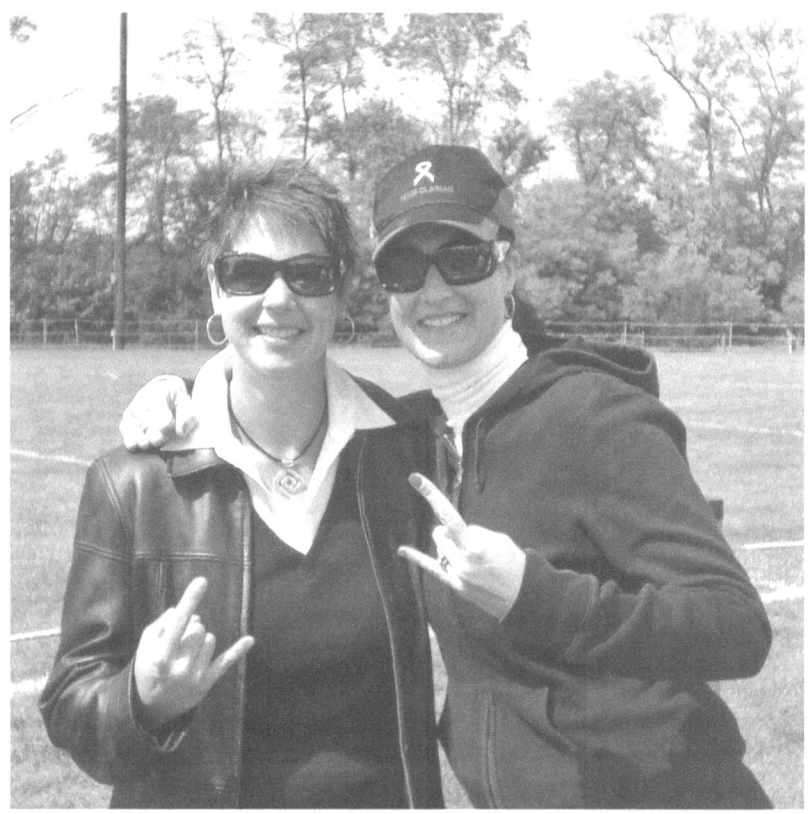

Lindsey and I about two hours before I shaved my head. This was the short hair cut I got in preparation for chemo. I also dyed my hair fire red for effect.

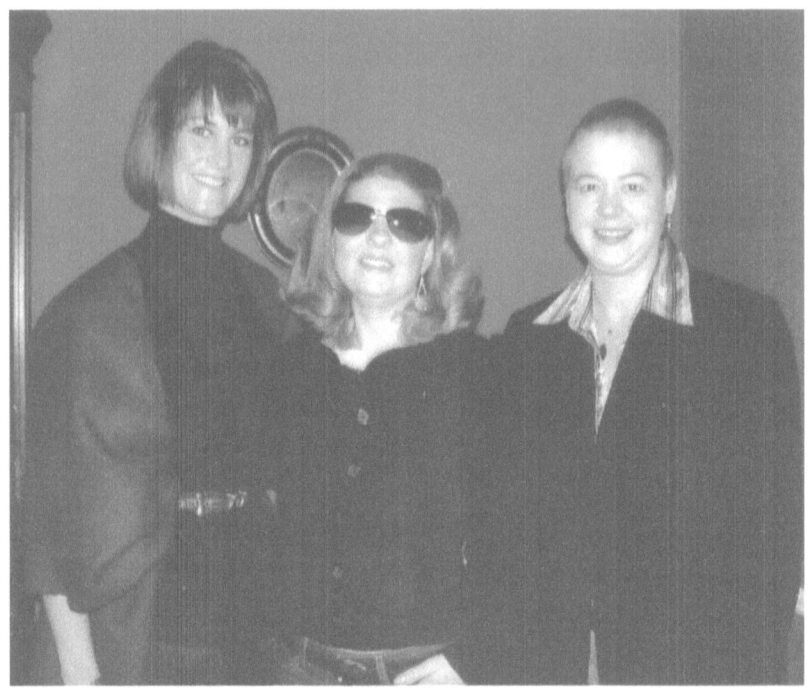

"My partying is getting in the way of my disease." From left to right: Lindsey, Ginger and myself. This was four days prior to surgery and we were going out for my last hurrah. My hair was coming back from chemo. You can see the weight I gained during chemo. Ginger was in the height of her myasthenia gravis. She is not wearing shades to be cool, but to hide her drooping eyelids.

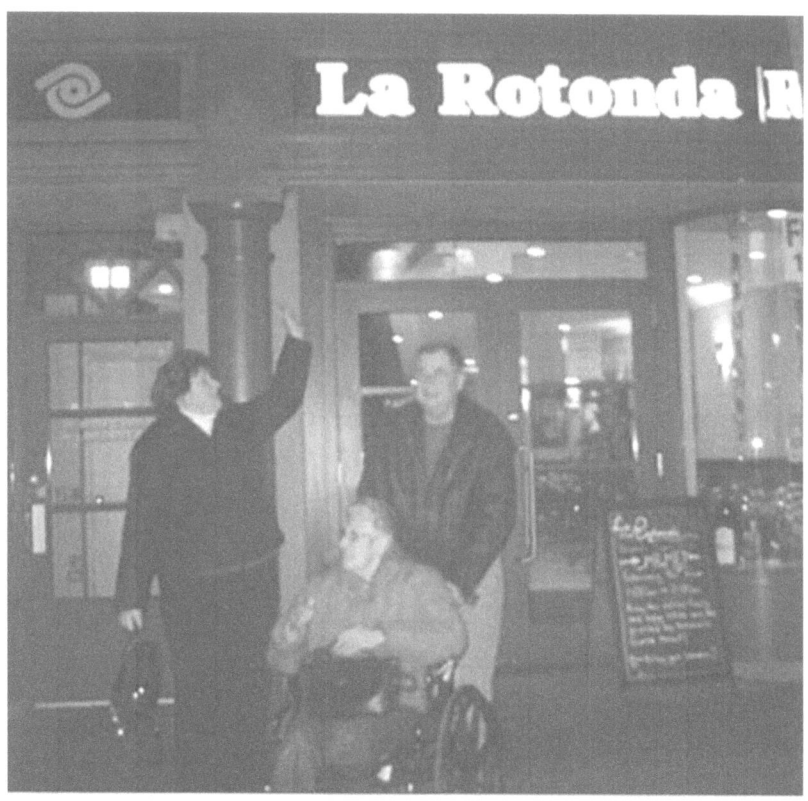

The drunkards rolling my mom back up the hill back home. She is not pleased.

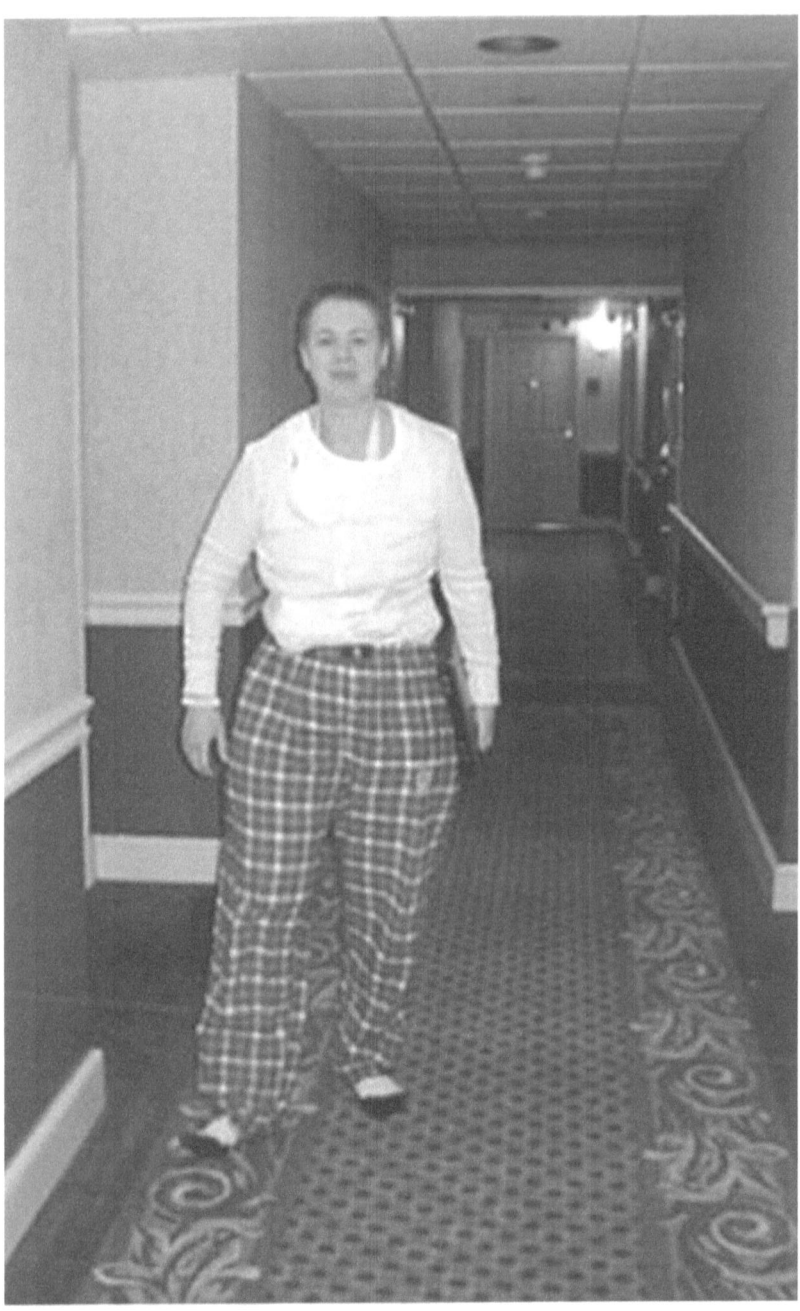

My first walk down the hallway at the senior assisted living facility. All those lumps in the front are the eight drains strategically placed.

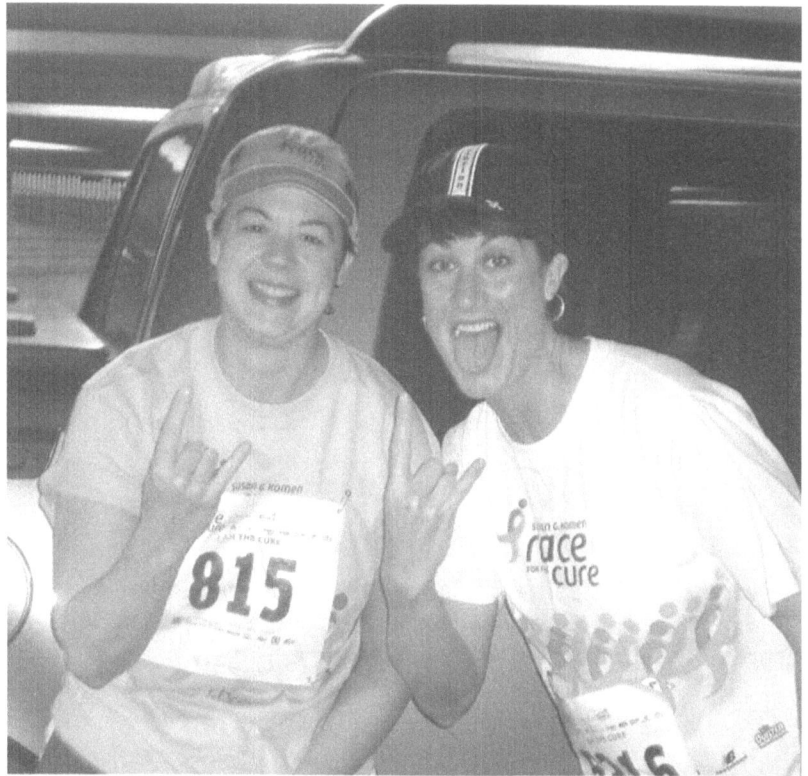

Lindsey and I getting ready to run Race for the Cure. This was just three months after my mastectomy and reconstruction surgery. Can you tell we like to make the Rock and Roll sign in all our pictures?

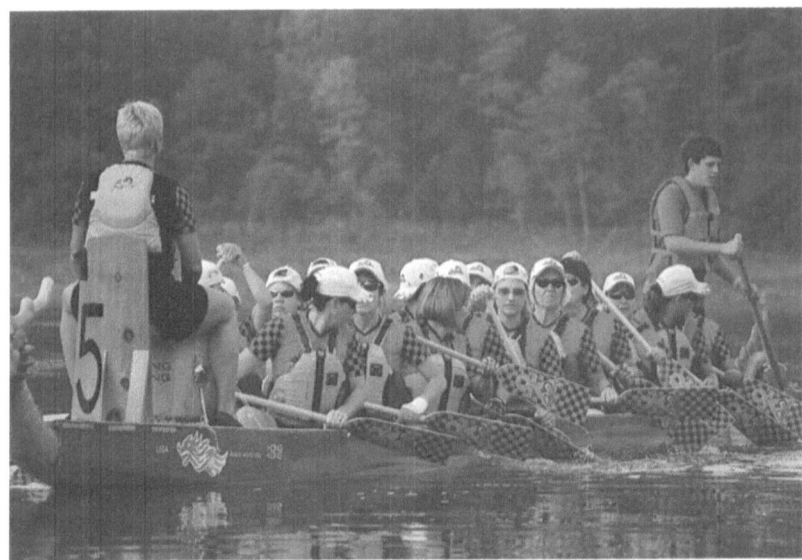

My dragon boat team getting ready to race. I am the serious one with the hat on backwards with the shades towards the front of the boat. I take competing very seriously!

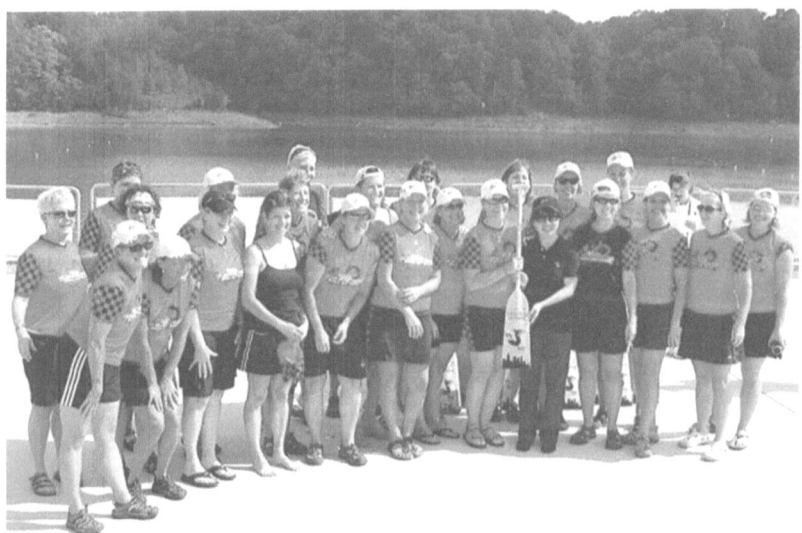

The Indy SurviveOars after a race. I am in the front row, 5th from the left. My team is awesome and I am proud to call myself a member.

Questions and/or Advice You May Want to Take to Your Various Appointments

THESE QUESTIONS ARE BY NO means comprehensive. Remember to bring a list of all medications, including vitamins, and a fairly comprehensive medical history to all your appointments. It will save you the headache of trying to remember everything. An important thing to remember is that information will be parsed out in steps. No one visit will tell you everything you want to know.

The mammogram:

Any mention of unusual results, calcium deposits or having to return for additional imaging should prompt you to ask the following:

1. If this is not your first mammogram, ask if the image compares to previous visits.
2. I would insist on an orthogonal technique if requested to come back in to take more images. In other words, if the technician is only planning to take additional angles by mammography, insist on an ultrasound at a minimum.
3. Remember that more than likely, there will not be complete resolution that day to what the images mean. Have some patience.

The Biopsy:

Okay, they want to sample the lump.

1. No matter what they tell you, take someone with you.

2. Before going to the biopsy, ask the doctor if the procedure will be performed in the office or in an OR setting—under mac-sedation.

3. If you are having the procedure performed in the office, ask about their numbing technique. Ask if you start to feel pain if they can stop and numb more or give you a mild sedative. Remember that you may be receiving a local anesthetic mixed with adrenaline.

The Phone Call:

So the phone is ringing and you hear those dreaded words, "You have cancer."

1. You may want to think about this event ahead of time and only give the doctor a phone number that you will answer in a safe environment, so that you are free to react in any manner which you choose. You do not know how you will react. The human mind is not predictable, so unless you are a Zen master of self control, I highly recommend just having them return calls to your home phone.

2. Ask when is the soonest you can come in and consult with the doctor.

3. Now is not the time to probe for information. They will not give it to you over the phone.

4. Contact someone you are close to. You may wait to do this, but at some point in the near future, I would recommend calling someone. You should not be alone because your imagination may begin to get wild.

The Diagnosis:

You have your appointment with your general surgeon to discuss your results.

1. Bring someone along. The amount of information, no matter how adept you believe you are to absorbing facts, there will

be things that you may miss. It is beneficial to have a second person there to verify what you were told, help ask questions that you may not think about and to provide emotional support.

2. Ask if they know the type of cancer. They should know this.

3. Ask to have your pathology slides sent to a second laboratory for verification. You should get a second opinion because errors have been made before. You may have to make the request yourself, but you are entitled to having a second opinion. This may also cost you a small amount of money.

4. At this visit, your doctor will discuss what they believe is the next steps for a course of treatment. Remember that this visit is with your general surgeon. The surgeon does not manage your cancer treatment. The general surgeon will, however, manage the preliminary tests required before treatment begins. You will want to get all of these tests completed prior to seeing an oncologist.

5. Ask if the doctor recommends an oncologist. Find out if he has worked with the oncologist before.

6. The doctor will not know anything at this point about how invasive the cancer is. They cannot answer the question you most want to ask, "Has it spread?" They also cannot answer what caused it.

7. If for any reason during this consultation, you are not comfortable with what the doctor is telling you, if you are not meshing with the doctor or if you know that you want to be treated somewhere else, you are within your right to seek out treatment from another physician. You are not bound to this doctor. You must do what is right for you. You are putting your life in this person's hands and you will be seeing this person often. The relationship with you and your doctor is key to believing in your treatment.

Hell Week:

Mentally you are a wreck. As I said in the narrative, this is the hardest time of cancer, believe it or not. This week is a whirlwind of visits to one random testing lab after another with no end in sight and no game plan.

1. Remember that all of the people you are dealing with are technicians specializing in operating that particular instrument. Sure, they probably know what they are looking at, but they are not allowed to give you information, no matter how much you beg and plead. Your general surgeon and oncologist will get the results.

2. Do not over interpret body language from the technician, any surplus clicking, extra pictures, etc.

3. Make sure you understand what you need to do to prepare for the test: whether you can eat beforehand, if you have to drink a bunch of water, drink a dye, etc. You do not want to take the time to show up only to have to reschedule.

4. You do not necessarily need a buddy for your tests, unless you want the support. Most do not involve any sedation or pain.

The Oncologist:

You have gone through the battery of tests and now have an appointment with your oncologist. This is the appointment where you will get a lot of information.

1. Take someone. I took two people, and let me tell you the amount of information was such that everyone missed something.

2. Take notes. Now the game plan begins and you want to be sure to capture all aspects of the plan. This helps you mentally transition from a victim to an active role in your treatment plan.

3. Do not be afraid to stop the doctor and ask for clarification.

4. Ask if you will receive chemotherapy.

5. If you are to receive chemo, ask about the timing of the therapy—right away or down the road.

6. Some doctors may want to perform a lumpectomy or mastectomy before any treatment. Ask for the rationale.

7. If you are to receive chemo, ask if you will be getting a port/central line to facilitate treatment. A port is recommended so that your veins do not get trashed. Ask about the timing of inserting the port relative to your chemo treatment.

8. If you are to receive chemo, a treatment plan will be given to you—type of drugs and how often. A list of side effects should be given to you. Note that the list is comprehensive and lists everything under the sun. Realize that chemo affects everyone differently.

9. If you are to receive chemo, you should be given a prescription for a wig at this appointment. Ask for recommendations for local shops that cater to cancer patients. Insurance should pay for a portion of the wig.

10. If you are to receive chemo, you may be told that you will receive a Neulasta® shot after treatment. Ask if you have to receive the shot in the office or if you can do this at home. This all depends on your insurance company's preference. It is more convenient to perform the shot at home from the perspective of one less visit to the chemo lounge and more waiting around. If you are given a prescription, make sure to fill it at the hospital as most local pharmacies do not carry this item.

11. You will be assigned a clinical nurse who will be your day-to-day point of contact for the duration of your treatment. Ensure that you get all of that individual's contact information. Any issues you have during treatment, this is your first point of contact to get the assistance you need, like prescriptions to treat side effects.

Chemotherapy:

You are getting chemo. Chemo day is not a fun one, but if you come prepared for the action, you can minimize your angst. The routine for myself for chemo was as follows. First I saw the oncologist for a check-up. This may have been the most agonizing part as I had to wait sometimes in upwards of two hours. He was worth waiting for! The doctor will perform a physical exam, including measurement of the tumor if it is at the surface. This is the time to be honest with how you are feeling. Following the exam, blood is drawn. Your platelets and white cell count must be at a certain level in order for you to receive chemo. Be prepared for the idea that you may not receive treatment that day, if your body is not bouncing back as it should.

1. You should be given a numbing cream to put on your skin over your port prior to anyone accessing it for blood draws or chemo. The problem is that if you cannot predict thirty minutes out from any of these events, the cream is not very helpful. I can attest that the numbing cream did not help me. Port access without the cream is no more painful than getting your veins jabbed.

2. When your port is accessed, they will flush with Heparin® and saline. The Heparin® may leave a funky medicinal taste in your mouth. It only lasts for a few seconds, but is a normal experience.

3. When you are scheduled for chemo, you will receive your doctor's appointment time, then your chemo time. Do not panic if you do not make your chemo time because of potential delays at the oncologist before. They are accustomed to this and you will get in for treatment, even at the end of the day.

4. Definitely have someone take you and bring things to do. Otherwise you will be subjected to the random entertainment that may or may not be provided. I found it beneficial to rotate who took me. It allows others to participate in your treatment and does not burden one person with taking a day out of their life every few weeks. The variety brings a source of entertainment, if nothing else.

5. Bring drinks and snacks that you like. It will be a long day.

6. I highly recommend if you are going to receive Adriamycin to take the nurse up on the offer to chew ice during the infusion. This helped me reduce mouth sores post treatment.

7. When you get home, pay attention to your body. I would nap for about an hour, then eat and exercise if I could.

Remember chemo does not have to equal being sick. I found the more activity I could stand, the better I felt.

8. Ask your oncologist about medications you can take with chemo. If you have allergies, for example, your oncologist will recommend what medication you should take for them. If you take herbal supplements, there will be some that you will not be allowed to take, especially if they contain hormones. I took vitamins, but only after clearing them with my oncologist.

9. As chemo progresses, you will become more tired. Stay in tune with your body requirements. Take a nap. If you do not, you will wear down very easily and could be susceptible to illness.

10. Towards the end of your chemo treatment regimen, ask about the plans for the port. Sometimes it is left in until surgery and removed then. You can have it taken out before then, especially if it is bothering you.

Plastic Surgeon:

Depending on the recommendation from your oncologist and general surgeon on whether you will receive a lumpectomy or a mastectomy, it will be the course of action. Let me say that you should see a plastic surgeon several months in advance of the end of your treatment. Doctors do not like to wait more than a couple of months after the end of treatment before removal of the tumor.

1. Get a feeling on whether you will need radiation or not. The need for radiation will dictate your plastic surgery options. You will not absolutely know until surgery where a biopsy of the lymph nodes occurs whether you will require radiation, but you can get a general sense from your oncologist and general surgeon beforehand.

2. Start with your general surgeon to get recommendations for plastic surgeons they have worked with in the past. The surgery is a team effort and you want your team to be in tune

with each other. However, you do not have to select their choice. It is all about who you feel comfortable with.

3. When you meet the plastic surgeon for the first time, you may want to take someone. Again, a lot of information will be given to you and having a second pair of ears will help disseminate the choices.

4. You do not have to commit to anything. You may want to go home and think about your options. Make sure to ask for all the options that are available.

5. Ask about the timing for surgery and the anticipated amount of recovery time post-surgery.

6. Ask about any restrictions that you will have after surgery.

7. If radiation is possibly in your future, prepare yourself for the fact that immediate reconstruction may not be an option.

8. I am an advocate of the DIEP if a mastectomy is your prognosis. Ask about it. If it is not offered in your local area, you can travel to have it done.

9. Be prepared for your first set of nudes—okay my first set, you may have had others taken…. Even if you do not commit to the surgeon, they may take 'before' pictures.

Surgery:

The big day has arrived. You will be given an extensive list of instructions.

1. Ask what time you will need to be at the hospital.

2. You will be told not to eat after midnight. You may ask if there are restrictions on what you can eat the night before.

3. Bring comfortable, loose clothing to wear home. I highly recommend getting a tank top to wear under your shirt, especially if you will be going home with drains still attached. It will help keep them from moving around.

4. You will need a kit. The kit needs to have a necklace to hold your drains, some tank tops—wife beaters for those familiar with the term,—pillows to put under your arms and a way to record your drain output. I will shamelessly plug my friend's

drain holders called the Tube-EZ—see the web link in the references section.

5. Ask about pain control. There are several different ways that your pain can be managed. Do not be afraid to let your caregivers know that you are in pain.

6. I will not sugar coat it: you will be in a world of hurt when you wake up. You may be nauseous. Your throat may be sore if you were intubated. Ask for ice chips. They will help.

7. Get up as soon as you can. You are not going to want to move, but moving is the key to getting better. The sooner you are up and about, the sooner you can go home.

8. Drink as much fluids as you can. If you have drains, you will be losing fluids there. Even if you are receiving an intravenous, supplement with lots of water.

9. Be cognizant of the last time you had a bowel movement. Do not wait a week before letting someone know you have not done your business. Magnesium citrate is a nasty, but effective tool for moving this activity along. The first bowel movement will not be pleasant, but it is a necessary evil.

10. About two weeks after surgery, you will want to begin performing the exercises that the doctor should have given you—ask for them before you leave the hospital. Make sure you do them so that scar tissue does not build up and cause a loss in your range of motion. Do not overdo it, since you just had major surgery. For recipients of the TRAM flap, hernias are a real concern.

11. Keep track of your drain output. A home nurse may be assigned to come and take care of your drains, or you may do it yourself. The drains will not come out until their production is low.

12. You will not want to wear anything but loose pants and shirts for a while. Plan your wardrobe accordingly.

13. When you go home, I recommend body pillows to help you sleep. You can roll over with the drains in with the pillows. Alternatively, you can build your own fortress with normal

pillows, but the body pillow would work the best, in my humble opinion.

Your Long Term Treatment:

This is for those who were diagnosed with an estrogen positive tumor, went through treatment and tumor removal and will now begin estrogen suppression therapy. At your first visit to the oncologist after surgery, you will be given your options on how to proceed.

1. Ask about the side effects of the medications. Tamoxifen has risks of other cancers associated with the medication. Aromatase inhibitors also have physical side effects that can become intolerable.

2. You may be put into menopause, or be there already. You cannot take herbal supplements that contain estrogen to help with the side effects. Antidepressants are an option to alleviate the hot flashes. There are side effects associated with these as well, so make sure to weigh all your options.

3. Let your doctor know immediately if you cannot tolerate the side effects. They can switch treatments.

4. Take your medication. Some individuals feel they are cancer free and do not want to commit to five years of more expense and feeling like crap, but in some cases, this course of medication is really your true treatment to prevent recurrence.

If you did not have both breasts removed, or only received a lumpectomy, you will also need to have routine imaging performed. Self exams are also very important to continue.

www.ingramcontent.com/pod-product-compliance
Lightning Source LLC
Chambersburg PA
CBHW020529290526
45786CB00002B/803